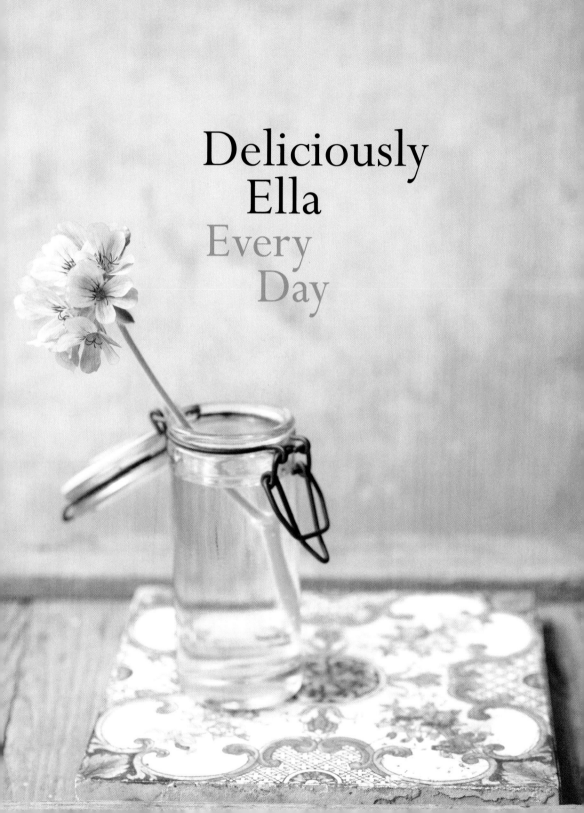

Deliciously
Ella

Every
Day

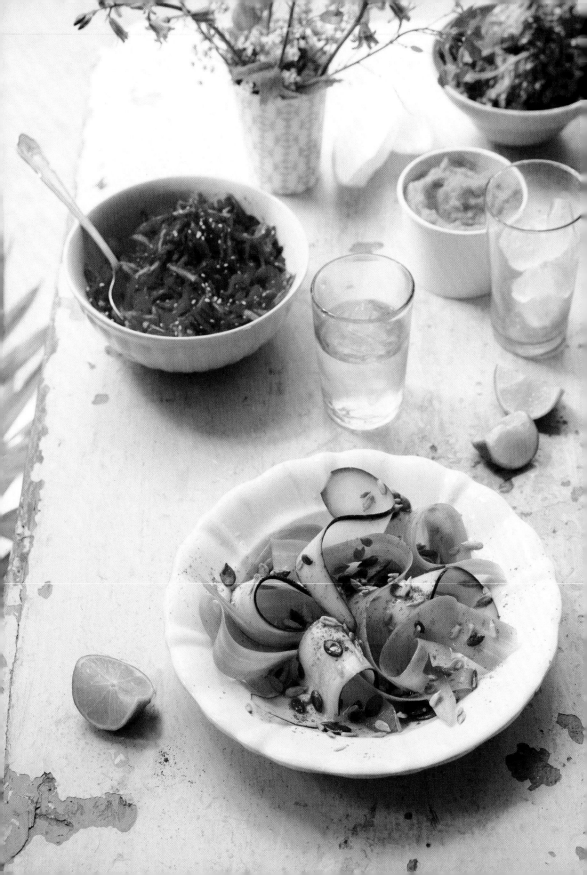

Deliciously Ella

Every Day

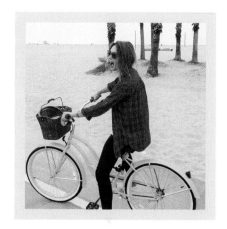

Quick and Easy Recipes
for Gluten-Free Snacks,
Packed Lunches and
Simple Meals

Ella
Woodward

SCRIBNER

New York   London   Toronto   Sydney   New Delhi

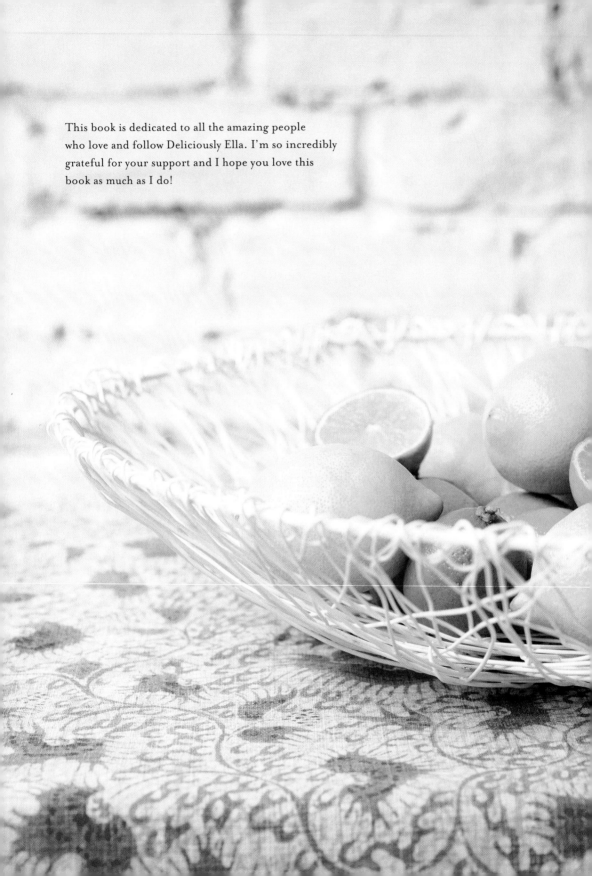

This book is dedicated to all the amazing people who love and follow Deliciously Ella. I'm so incredibly grateful for your support and I hope you love this book as much as I do!

CONTENTS

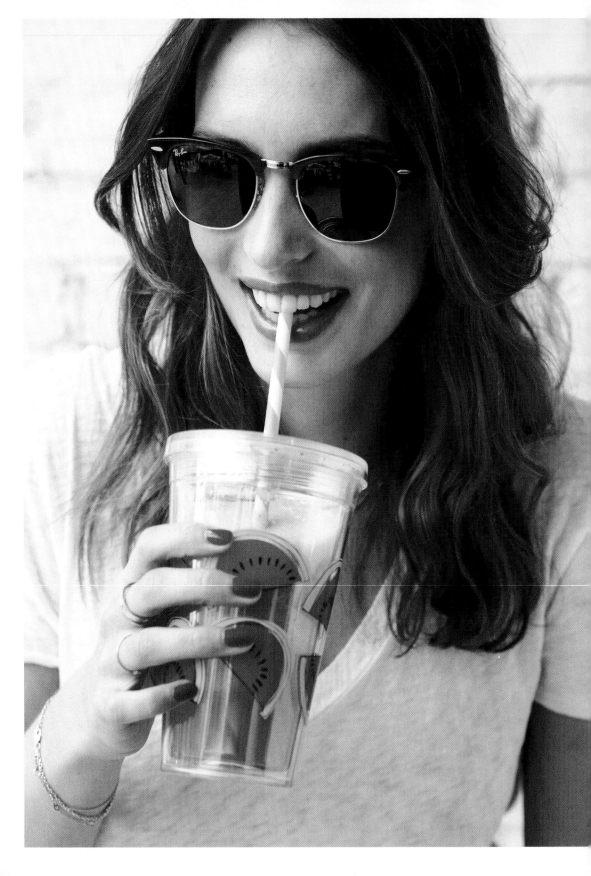

INTRODUCTION

Healthy living has totally transformed my life and I think it will transform yours, too. I changed my diet in January 2012 to try to heal a chronic illness called postural tachycardia syndrome. Overnight I adopted a natural, plant-based diet and said good-bye to gluten, dairy, refined sugar, processed food, additives and meat. It was a dramatic change, especially as I had mainly lived off pesto pasta, candy and chocolate up until then . . .

It took a while for the diet to work but, over the course of eighteen months, I got better, came off all my medications and realized that living a healthy life made me happier and healthier than I ever had been before. It wasn't an easy journey, though, and one of the things I found hardest was learning how to eat well when I was really busy and pushed for time. So that's the purpose of this book: to share my tips and tricks to help you build the Deliciously Ella way of eating into your everyday life, so that you can look and feel your best, too. Taking care of yourself is much easier than you may think and, with a little organization, you can eat amazing, nourishing food all week long, all year round.

To me, the most important thing about healthy eating is that the food is always both delicious and do-able. Nourishing your body with goodness needs to fit into your existing lifestyle and not feel like a crazy, overwhelming task. I want to show you how to throw together simple, natural ingredients in just a few minutes to create a fantastic meal and also to help you plan better, so you can always have an awesome, healthy option available to eat throughout the day, whether you're at home or not.

In this book I'll introduce you to more than one hundred of my staple dishes, the things that I cook time and time again and the recipes that always make me happy. I've tried to keep things as quick and easy as possible, with minimal preparation time, so hopefully you'll fall in love with the taste and ease of each creation and, over time, these wonderful recipes will become a part of your life.

I'm going to share my speedy weekday dinners, from almond butter quinoa, to the best baked sweet potato with garlic mushrooms, to pasta arrabbiata, to new-style nori rolls with avocado cream. We'll also explore easy bigger meals, either to serve to all your friends and family, or to be frozen to provide the healthiest "ready meals," such as black bean burgers, my favorite sweet potato cakes and chickpea quinoa and turmeric curry.

I've also included a healthy eating on-the-go section, which will spice up your work or school lunches so much that everyone around you will have serious food envy! Plus we'll go through the best easy breakfasts (think overnight oats, five-minute porridge and maple chia pots), my go-to simple sweet treats (coconut and raspberry mousse, cacao oat and raisin cookies and the best hot chocolate) and lots of amazing salads. So, by the time you finish this book, you'll have a whole new range of straightforward go-to meals that will keep you inspired and energized every day!

CHANGING YOUR EATING HABITS

Shifting toward a more plant-based way of life is pretty exciting; it opens up a whole new world of delicious ingredients, amazing tastes and unique textures and truly makes you feel fabulous from the inside out. But I know that it's not the easiest adjustment and that it throws up its own challenges.

For me, the biggest hurdle was losing the meals that I had relied on almost every day—pesto pasta, cereal, smoked salmon bagels, lasagne and chicken stir-fry—and having to find alternatives. It can be hard at first when old favorites suddenly vanish. Don't worry: you're absolutely not alone in staring at the supermarket shelves having no idea what to buy or what to do with your purchases once you get them home. In fact, it seems to be an issue for almost everyone I've spoken to who is changing to a plant-based diet. Don't panic! I am here to help.

Another issue I found was that I got stuck in a serious food rut. While I absolutely adore food, and eating is probably my favorite pastime, I admit I am naturally a lazy cook. I like fast, easy meals that taste

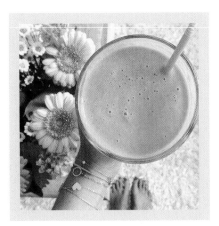

wonderful but require minimal preparation, chopping and washing up! This disposition, combined with the fact that I didn't know what to cook or how to cook it, meant that I ate the same thing almost every day for the first few months of my plant-based life! Everything tasted good, but I was bored with the lack of variety, which meant that I didn't truly appreciate how amazing plant-based food really is. I only actually fell in love with this way of eating when I pushed myself to try new things, and in doing so I discovered a whole world of rainbow goodness and—even more importantly—I realized that cooking awesome, healthy, varied meals every day was incredibly easy, which is why I wanted to write this book for you.

FINDING BALANCE

While I hope to persuade you to eat more plant-based goodness, I absolutely don't expect you to only eat this way and I know that almost no one becomes a gluten-free, sugar-free veggie overnight! I'm not here to preach or to make anyone feel guilty about enjoying pizza, cheese and chocolate cake; after all, the Deliciously Ella way of eating and living is all about positivity. Instead, I want to make it as easy as possible for you to combine Deliciously Ella recipes with any other kinds of food.

I believe that we should all try to nourish our bodies with plant-based food when we're at home: for weekday breakfasts, work lunches, Tuesday nights when you're eating in the kitchen . . . that sort of thing. These are the times it makes sense to eat the Deliciously Ella way, as you're not having to conform to social conventions at restaurants or eat someone else's food in their home, so you don't have to worry about being rude or different from everybody else.

Eating my way at home means your body has a healthy foundation, so you can go for dinner with friends, order what you want and savor

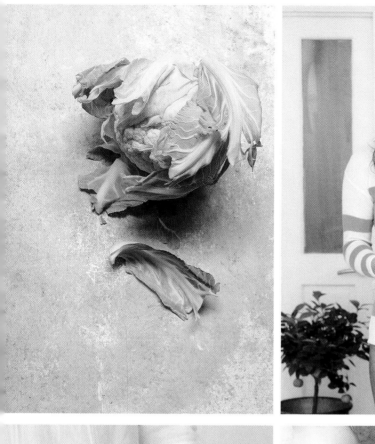
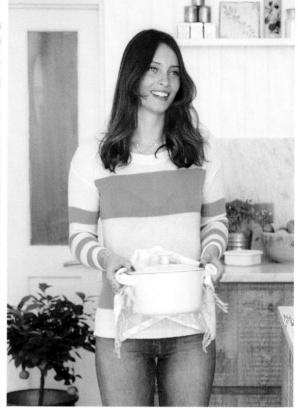
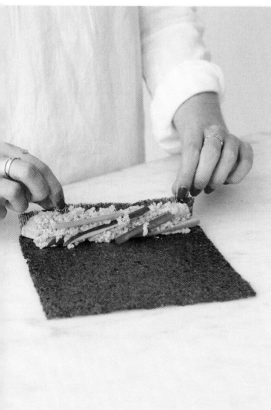
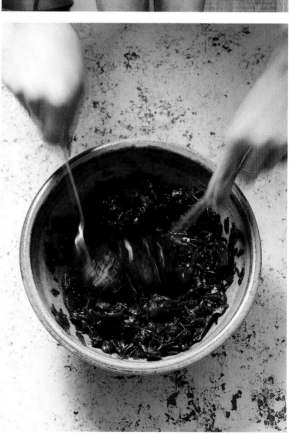

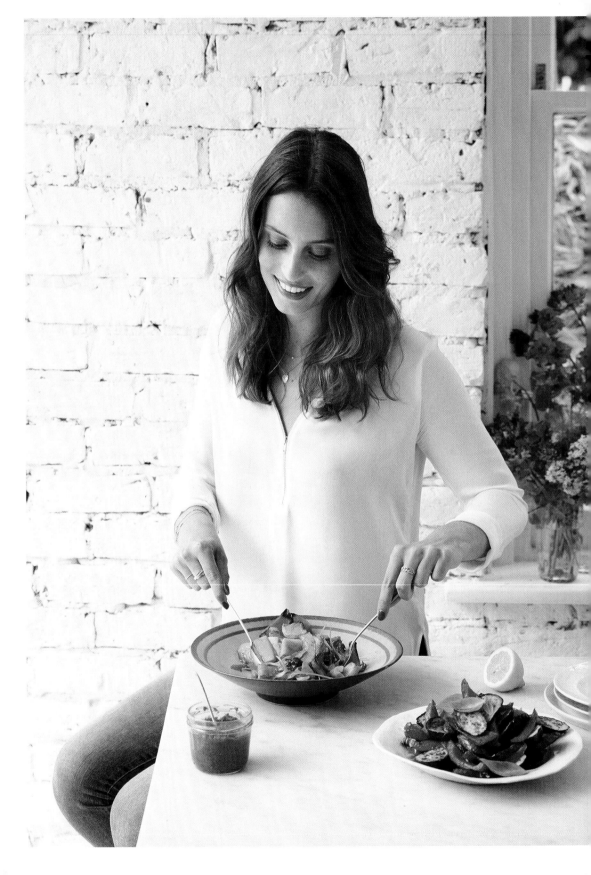

it: if you love pizza, order an amazing pizza; if you love cookies, get the best cookie and actually think about and appreciate each bite as you eat. This is the balance I'm talking about: healthy moderation. It will make healthy eating so much more accessible rather than trying to eat this way all the time right from the outset. It also means that trying to be super-healthy won't take over your life and stress you out when you don't know what to order from a not-so-healthy restaurant menu. It's important that this balance feel relaxed and easy, rather than you feeling compelled to do a juice cleanse because you ate one too many pieces of chocolate cake the night before!

However, if you want to eat this way all the time, as I do, then of course that's amazing and something I would encourage. The vital thing is to find what works for you. For lots of people this means just one meal a day based on the Deliciously Ella philosophy, for others it means eating fifty percent plant-based and fifty percent traditional food, and for a few (myself included) it means always eating this way, because you love it. It doesn't matter which category you fall into, we all have to start somewhere! Besides, it's so important to know that every change you make is beneficial to your body. Each time you add a portion of veggies, whole grains or fruits to your meal, you're doing an amazing thing for yourself.

WHERE TO START

My advice would be to experiment with one or two plant-based recipes each week, say on a weekday evening when you're at home. Try this for a few weeks, then start to add in a couple of healthy breakfasts. You can choose breakfast recipes that are made the night before so, on the night you cook your Deliciously Ella dinner, you can also make an awesome breakfast for the next day. Once you're finding the breakfast

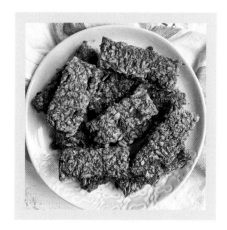

and dinner options fun and easy, then start switching up your lunches to incorporate some of the suggestions in my on-the-go chapter, or try serving some of the salad or dessert recipes at a dinner party.

There's no rush. Taking small steps often leads to the best outcome, as you won't feel overwhelmed by change and start craving everything you're used to eating. To stop this from happening, you can also combine Deliciously Ella meals with your old favorites —add roast salmon to your quinoa, parmesan to your pasta and fries to your veggie burger, for instance—if this gets you trying new plant-based recipes then it's wonderful and nothing to feel bad about!

You'll find that the more you start to eat this way the better you'll feel and I promise it will become quite addictive; waking up feeling amazing every day is honestly the best thing and, once that starts to happen, you'll never go back to eating the way you did before! Your taste buds will also start to change and, over the course of a few months, medjool dates will start to taste like the sweetest things on earth, so you won't feel a need for lots of refined sugar either.

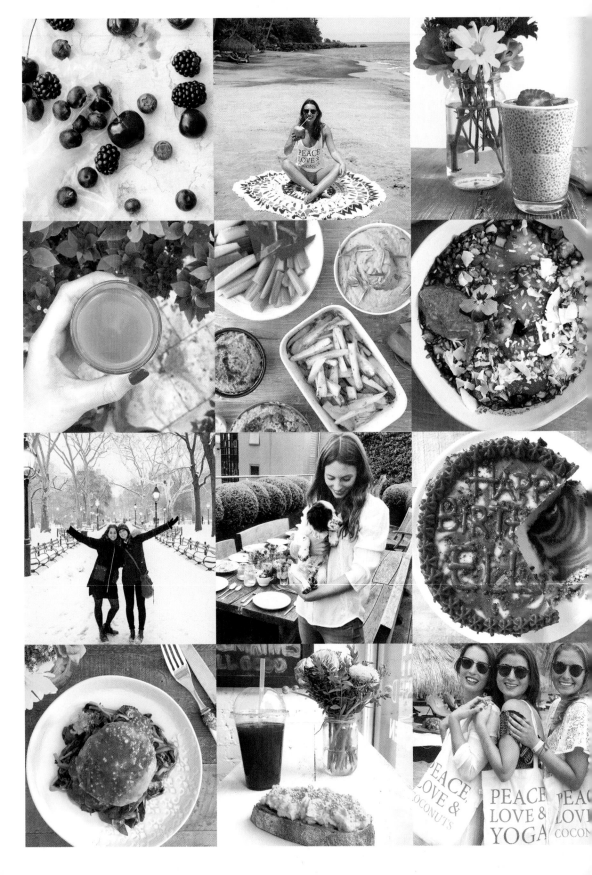

HOW TO LIVE A DELICIOUSLY ELLA LIFESTYLE

Before we get into the ins and outs of how to be organized and stay healthy when you're really busy, I quickly want to run you through my "ten commandments" for living a healthy, happy life. I know that food can be a complicated, emotional topic for people and that eating healthily can become obsessive and compulsive in the way that lots of diets can, when in reality it should just be a fun, easy, flexible component of your life. So I hope that the points below will guide you to a state of being where you can love anything and everything that you eat.

Enjoy your food—no matter what you're eating, whether it's kale or pizza, love every bite and savor each flavor. Food should always be fun.

Don't look at healthy eating as a "diet"—it's a lifestyle and an awesome way of living, so don't deprive or starve yourself, as this won't make you happy or healthy. Remember, we're not counting calories or measuring portion sizes.

Open your mind—try new things and be flexible about your existing views on healthy eating. You'll find healthy food is so much better than bland salads and you'll enjoy it far more.

Balance is everything!—find what works for you, set realistic goals and be happy with them.

Be organized—take a little time every week to stock your fridge with nourishing ingredients, snacks and meals, so you always have something delicious on hand to eat.

Treat your body with respect—it is a beautiful, amazing thing that needs to be listened to. If you're full, stop eating; if you're hungry, have a snack; if you have digestive issues, examine your diet. Your body knows what it needs, you just need to learn to hear what it's saying.

Eat a rainbow—try to make each meal as colorful as you can. Not only will this give you the best array of vitamins and minerals, it will also make your plate look more beautiful and appetizing. We all eat with our eyes first, so it will make your meal more delicious, too.

Don't feel guilty—if all you want is chocolate cake, then eat a slice and enjoy it. Don't binge-eat it and feel guilty afterward, and absolutely don't restrict what you eat the next day as a result. Remember: no one is perfect!

Get creative—enjoy experimenting in the kitchen with new recipes and ingredients, adapt them as you like and don't be afraid to try different things.

Slow down—take a minute to enjoy what you're eating and don't inhale your food. It takes about twenty minutes for your brain to register how full you are, plus you won't appreciate how great the food is if you don't take the time to think about it while you eat each bite.

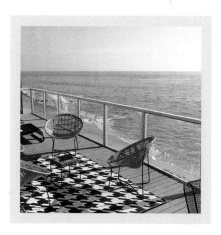

HOW TO PREPARE IN ADVANCE

The boring news is that staying healthy is all about organization; I know that doesn't sound exciting but it's so true. I'll write more about getting organized in the on-the-go chapter, but for now I want to run through a few of the little things you should keep in your kitchen to help you with the organizational part.

Most importantly you'll need lots of great containers; they will make all the difference to how good your food tastes and how long it stays fresh. It also means you can easily store food to take away with you, so you can just grab a container of goodness from the fridge, put it in your bag and bring it along to wherever you have to be. So what exactly do you need?

Glass jars with lids—my favorite storage items. They make everything look so pretty and it feels so much nicer picking up a beautiful jar than a plastic box! You can buy really cheap small glass jars online, or you can be super-eco-friendly and recycle old jars, which is what I do: my kitchen is filled with old tahini, almond butter and honey jars! Recycling jars also means you'll have a wonderful range of shapes and sizes, so you'll always have the perfect jar for your creation. I use jars for my breakfasts all the time as they're perfect for holding smoothies, overnight oats and chia pots. I also use big jars to store my dry goods, mainly my nuts, grains and seeds.

Airtight food containers—your food needs to be kept airtight, as this stops it from going bad or losing flavor. Airtight, waterproof plastic boxes may not look as beautiful as glass jars, but they're a total lifesaver when it comes to transporting your lunch. I keep my on-the-go lunches and leftover meals in these boxes in the fridge, plus I use them to store brownies, cookies, energy balls and pretty much everything else! You can buy them in all sizes and colors from almost everywhere.

Freezer bags—to be honest, these aren't super-exciting either, but they're very handy! They are the easiest way to store things in the freezer. Unlike plastic boxes, they take up very little space, so if you have a tiny freezer you should still be able to fit lots of bags on each shelf. I use them for portions of big batches of soup: I just take a bag out of the freezer and leave it in a bowl on the side to defrost for a few hours before I warm it up. Freezer bags are also great for storing slices of bread; as I don't normally get through a loaf in a week I keep half of it, ready-sliced, in the freezer, so I can just take a piece out when I want. I also store frozen fruit in bags, as it takes up less space.

Glass bottles with rubber seals—these are less important than the three items above, but still really helpful to have around. I use them to store my nut milks, smoothies and juices, as they keep the air out to help keep whatever I've made fresh. It's so important that the lid have a rubber seal around it, or air can get in and spoil what you've made. Again, these are readily available and really inexpensive.

OTHER EQUIPMENT

As well as the basics—grater, garlic crusher, kitchen scales and veggie peeler—a powerful blender is kind of essential and a food processor is useful as it means you can make more (especially when it comes to my soups, dips, dressings and smoothies). I've written at length about those in my first book, *Deliciously Ella*, so I won't go into detail here except to say that they're both worth investing in. I've tried to keep their usage to a minimum, though, so the recipes are achievable for everyone. And if you want to eat my zucchini noodles, a spiralizer would be handy and won't break the bank, but you can use a veggie peeler instead. If you're planning on making your own plant-based milks, you will also need a nut milk bag.

STORAGE

Again, I know this isn't the most scintillating topic, but knowing how to properly store dry goods, as well as your awesome meals, means that you'll get the most out of them.

STORING DRY GOODS

As I've said, I like using glass jars. I have shelves in my kitchen filled with almonds, cashews, quinoa, buckwheat, chickpeas, brown rice, chia seeds, cacao nibs, gluten-free pasta, oats and so on. It looks beautiful and it means you can see exactly what you have and how much of it is left. I find it's a more economical way of keeping food, as I don't go and buy more of something that I already have but couldn't see, plus it means that you don't have chickpeas and almonds spilling out of plastic packages everywhere!

I recycle small jars for things such as chia seeds or cacao nibs, and buy big rubber-sealed jars to keep bulk items, such as rice and pasta.

USING THE FRIDGE

This may sound like a totally ridiculous heading, I thought it was too when I first wrote it, as doesn't everyone know what a fridge is and how to use one? But if you're not

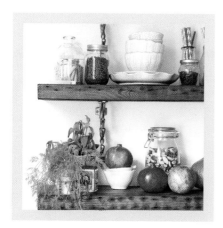

much of a cook, then there are a few tips that can help you. The first thing to note is that putting anything in the fridge will cause it to lose some flavor; the cold just does this to food. So when you're eating leftovers it's important to let them warm up, otherwise you won't enjoy them half as much. Either let them sit at room temperature for twenty minutes or so, or warm them in a pan with a little olive oil to remedy any dryness that has happened in the fridge. I do the same thing with any overnight breakfast recipe: I'll take it out as soon as I wake up, so that by the time I have showered, dressed and got ready for the day it will have warmed up enough to taste delicious.

I keep leftover meals that I'm going to eat within the next few days in the fridge; if I'm not going to eat them in this time frame, I'll put them in the freezer so they will keep for longer.

I don't put baked goods in the fridge as I find it changes their flavor too much. Instead, they go into airtight boxes at room temperature.

USING THE FREEZER

Again, this might sound like a mad heading, but there are a few tips that can be handy here. The first is that it's best to store as much as you can in freezer bags, as it saves so much room and you can see what you have, so you won't have a curry sitting in the freezer for a year . . .

The other important thing is that you can freeze almost anything! Whenever I have overripe fruit, I chop it up and throw it into a bag in the freezer. I'll do the same if I have too much spinach or kale, so I can use them frozen in my smoothies. It prevents waste and ensures that your drink is nice and cold.

If I have a frozen meal that I want to eat that evening, I take it out of the freezer when I leave the house in the morning and put it in the fridge to defrost; that way when I come home I can just put it straight in a pan to heat up, rather than dealing with a giant ice cube of stew!

The last thing to note is that food should only

be defrosted once, so just take the amount you need out of the freezer and leave the rest of the meal in there for another time. (This is why it's a good idea to freeze a meal in portions, rather than all in the same bag.)

SHOPPING LIST

As you go through the book you'll see that the same ingredients come up all the time. This overlap is deliberate, as it means your meals will be quicker and cheaper to prepare and you won't be spending lots of money on an ingredient that you'll only use in one recipe.

If you're totally new to this way of eating then it will be expensive to do an initial shop, to stock your cabinets with the items below; however, after this your meals should cost very little, as all you'll need to buy are a few fresh ingredients. If you're making Bircher muesli, for example, all you'll need to buy are apples and, if you're making the lentil and eggplant pasta, all you'll need are eggplants and red peppers.

The fresh ingredients for my recipes are available anywhere in the world, so if your cabinets are stocked with everything else it will always be easy to make these recipes. I tend to shop for all the pantry ingredients listed here online, as I find it much easier: you often get better deals and won't have to spend ages running around supermarkets to get dinner together, which is good in terms of saving time. Also, some smaller supermarkets may not stock items such as brown rice flour, coconut oil and chia seeds (though, these days, more and more of them do, which is amazing). If your cabinets are stocked with everything you need to make a wonderfully healthy and very delicious meal, then you're much more likely to actually make it, rather than resorting to a bowl of cereal or ordering takeout.

I find the internet is normally the best place to get great deals on health foods, so I normally order from there. Even though your first shop will be expensive, everything you buy will last for ages, so it won't go to waste . . . you never need to worry about your quinoa, tamari and maple syrup going off! I've talked more about the cost of eating this way in the Big-Batch Cooking chapter, so I won't go into too much detail about it here, but just trust me: it's so worth investing in your health.

DRY INGREDIENTS

Buckwheat groats
Cacao powder (raw)
Chia seeds
Flour (brown rice and buckwheat)
Hemp seeds
Noodles (buckwheat)
Nuts (almonds, cashews, hazelnuts, pecans)
Oats
Pasta (brown rice)
Pine nuts
Pumpkin seeds
Puy lentils
Quinoa
Rice (brown and short-grain brown)
Sesame seeds
Sunflower seeds

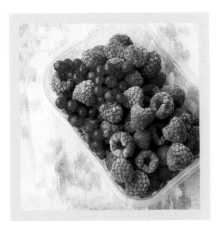

CANNED GOODS

Black beans
Cannellini beans
Chickpeas
Coconut milk
Tomatoes (chopped)

CONDIMENTS/WET INGREDIENTS

Almond butter
Apple cider vinegar
Coconut oil
Miso paste
Olive oil
Sesame oil
Sun-dried tomatoes
Tahini
Tamari
Tomato paste

FRIDGE/FREEZER

Frozen peas
Plant-based milk

HERBS AND SPICES

Basil (fresh)
Cayenne pepper
Chili flakes
Cilantro (fresh)
Cinnamon (ground)
Coriander (ground)
Cumin (ground)
Ginger (ground and fresh root)
Mixed herbs/herbes de Provence
Paprika
Turmeric
Vanilla pods and powder

SWEETENERS

Dates (ideally medjool)
Honey (raw)
Maple syrup
Raisins

On top of these, there are a few fresh items that I buy every week as they are used in so many of my recipes. I often have an online delivery arranged for these on a Sunday evening, so my fridge is stocked with goodness all week and I'm inspired to make lots of healthy meals.

FRESH FRUIT AND VEG

Apples
Avocados
Bananas
Beets
Blueberries
Butternut squash
Carrots
Cauliflower
Cucumbers
Eggplant
Garlic
Kale
Lemons and limes
Mangoes
Mushrooms
Parsnips
Peppers
Potatoes
Raspberries
Spinach
Strawberries
Sweet potatoes
Tomatoes
Zucchini

Food healed me and made me feel better and more energized than ever before. Now, I want to show you how exciting it can be to eat a plant-based diet and also to inspire you with some of my fabulous recipes.

Let's get cooking!

BREAKFAST

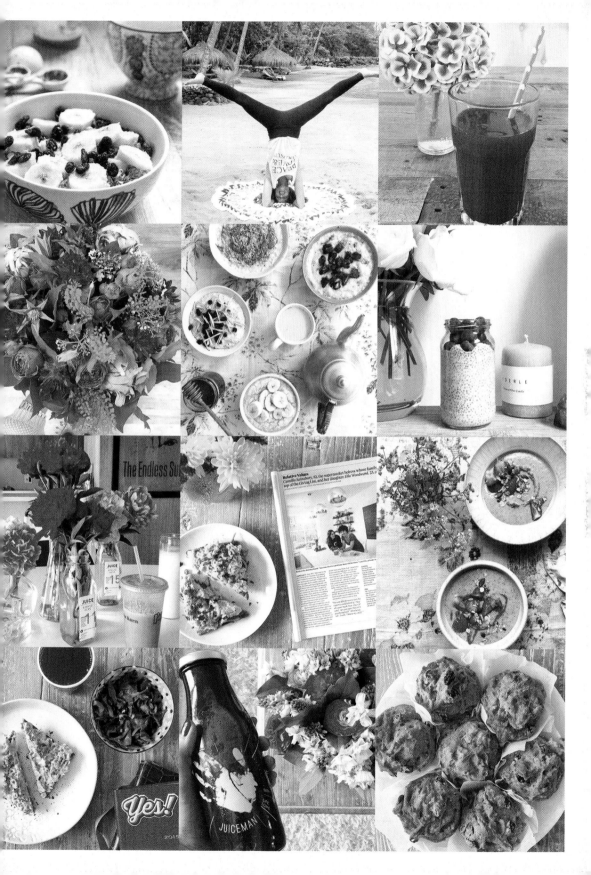

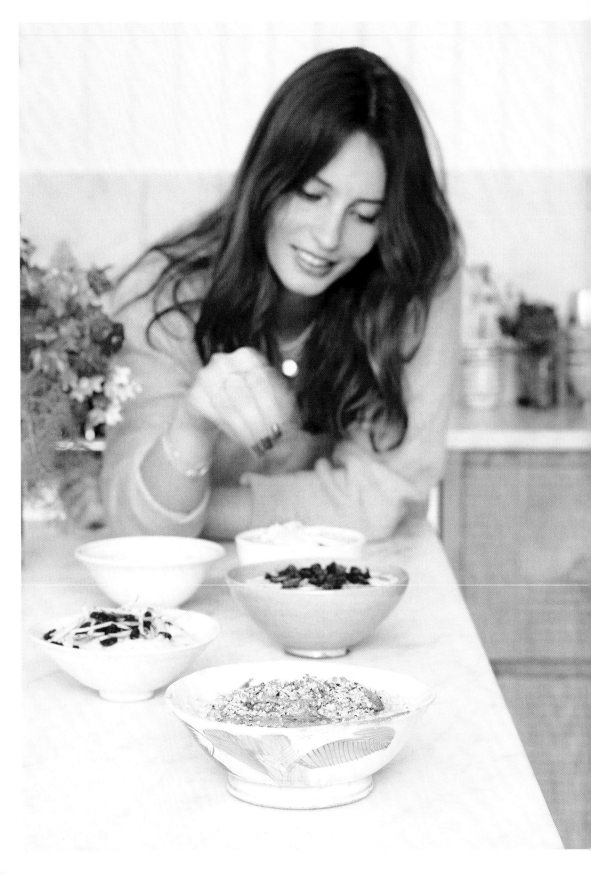

BREAKFAST

Without a doubt, breakfast is my favorite meal of the day; I absolutely love it! As soon as I wake up, I start dreaming of some delicious creation and it immediately gets me out of bed. In the winter I love a big bowl of piping hot porridge topped with cinnamon and sweet medjool dates, or warm slices of Zucchini Banana Bread spread with a thick layer of almond butter (pages 32 and 40). During the summer I like something cooler and lighter, so I get excited about my Maple Chia Pots, creamy Bircher Muesli and vibrant smoothies (pages 25, 30 and 47–51). Sound good?

I know you're probably thinking you would never have the time to make any of these as you rush out the door in the morning, but I'll let you in on a secret: you really do. I've created this book with busy people in mind and almost all the recipes in this chapter take less than ten minutes to make in the morning, or they're made the night before so they're ready for you to grab and go first thing. And don't worry, none of them is complicated or requires you to spend hours whisking or baking. Plus, to make life even easier, you can make a few servings of each at a time, so you only have to make breakfast twice a week, which is awesome as you'll have a fridge full of delicious breakfasts ready to go!

Making the decision to eat well in the morning is so important, as it sets the tone for your whole day. It's really worth getting up ten minutes earlier than usual so you can create a beautiful, nourishing breakfast that will give you the physical and emotional energy you need to have a great day.

On a physical level, eating a delicious, healthy breakfast filled with an amazing array of vitamins, minerals, fiber, good fats and plant-based proteins means you will have all the energy you need to run around and do everything you have to do. The energy will be released slowly over a few hours, so you won't get sugar spikes or crashes. As a result, you'll feel balanced and stable and won't get any serious sugar cravings. Also, you will start to feel hungry gradually, a few hours after you've eaten, so you won't feel the need to instantly eat whatever is in front of you (which may derail your healthy eating plan), nor will your stomach start to growl. Instead, you'll simply begin to get excited about your lunch.

On an emotional level, eating a healthy breakfast gives you the mental strength to look after your body for the rest of the day, as you'll feel good about yourself. Eating a meal that doesn't make you feel bloated or lethargic an hour later is great, especially when it also helps you to get glowing skin, shiny hair and bright eyes. It's amazing knowing you're doing something that will make you look and feel your best. Once you've made that decision at breakfast, you'll most likely be inspired to continue on a positive path all day, probably eat a more nutritious lunch and dinner and just have a happier day all round. It also means that exercise and meditation will seem more appealing, as you'll feel balanced and motivated. All these things will increase your happiness and inspire you to eat more nourishing food: a very positive cycle that I recommend!

I know I'm pinning a lot on breakfast, but I do think that the way you start your day is often the way that you continue it, so do it right!

I admit that, even though breakfast is my favorite meal, I actually find that it can be the hardest to eat well at, and much harder than lunch and dinner. I've heard this from lots of other people, too, so if you feel the same, you're not alone. The problem is that "traditional" breakfasts—cereal, white bread, processed jams, pastries, orange juice from a carton—are full of gluten, dairy and sugar. They can be convenient and their packaging may try to sell you health claims but, trust me, none of them will start your day the right way. So I hope this chapter will steer you away from those kinds of foods and get you excited about a new "world of breakfast," full of fresh, whole ingredients that will have you buzzing with energy.

So, what should we eat for breakfast to get a happy glow? I love using simple, nourishing staples—what I call my "super-start ingredients"—oats, buckwheat groats, bananas, apples, avocados, chia seeds and plant-based milks such as cashew milk. I use these to make all my favorites: Sweet Beet Overnight Oats; Raw Buckwheat Bowls; Speedy Porridge; Carrot Cake Muffins; Chili-Avocado Toast and Banana Breakfast Bars, great for when you're on-the-go (pages 26, 28, 32, 35, 42 and 44).

MY FAVORITE BREAKFAST INGREDIENTS

First, I want to share a little more information with you on my super-start ingredients, so you'll know more about why you're using them and all the amazing things they can do for you.

Oats—delicious and amazingly versatile, these can be used in so many ways from porridge to smoothies, muffins, muesli and breakfast bars. They're really filling, too, as they contain incredible amounts of fiber, which helps keep you satisfied for hours and means you avoid blood sugar spikes and crashes, while also helping your digestive system to work more efficiently. As a result, you should have lots of energy all day. Be careful of the different types of oats out there! Quick-cooking oats are very thin and just take three or four minutes to cook; soaking them would turn them into mush. Extra-thick rolled oats take much longer to cook and will need much more liquid, so use standard rolled oats instead.

Gluten-free oats—there's some confusion out there, as you can buy gluten-free oats, which implies that regular oats do contain gluten . . . but they don't. Oats contain avenin, a protein that almost all coeliacs and gluten-intolerant people do well with. (It is possible to be sensitive to avenin, but this is different from gluten intolerance.) So what's the difference between regular and gluten-free oats? Regular oats are packaged in factories that also process gluten; so there is a risk of cross-contamination. Nevertheless, I advise buying regular oats, unless you suffer from coeliac disease, in which case it's best to be extra-careful. I have a very intense reaction to gluten, but I feel equally awesome after eating regular oats and gluten-free oats.

Buckwheat groats—if you're sensitive to oats, or just feel like something different, buckwheat is a great option. Despite the confusing name, buckwheat is a gluten-free grain (technically it's a seed, but it tastes and cooks like a grain). It's delicious in both cooked and raw porridge and, if you're sensitive to oats, you can adapt any of the quick-cooking oat recipes here to use buckwheat. Buckwheat is of course full of goodness, too, especially plant protein, which means it's fantastic for boosting morning energy levels.

Plant-based milks—a pretty essential breakfast ingredient used in almost every recipe in this chapter. There are lots of types: nut milks, such as almond, cashew and Brazil nut; oat milk; hemp milk; rice milk; coconut milk . . . the list goes on. I tend to use almond, cashew and oat milks as I like their tastes best. You'll find my Creamy Cashew Milk recipe in this chapter (page 53), while almond and oat milk recipes are in my first book. I prefer to make my own milks and really urge you to do the same, as almost all store-bought milks contain additives and sweeteners. The recipe list of the most popular almond milk brand reads: water, sugar, almonds (2%!), tri-calcium phosphate, sea salt, locust bean gum, gellan gum, emulsifier, vitamins. So there's more sugar in it than almonds and I'm not desperately excited to be drinking the other stuff either. Homemade milks are easy to make and so much better for you.

Bananas—my favorite breakfast fruit. These go into delicious porridge, Zucchini Banana Bread, are often a topping for toast and make perfect smoothies (pages 32, 40, 42 and 47–51). They add great sweetness and a creamy texture that I love. They're also full of fiber, vitamins and minerals, especially potassium (great for maintaining healthy blood pressure and preventing cramping after exercise).

Apples—another great breakfast fruit. Like bananas, they add a beautiful sweetness to any recipe, so I use them a lot. I love them grated into porridge, mixed into my Sweet Beet Ovenight Oats and Bircher Muesli (pages 26 and 30) and used as a purée in my bread and muffins. Apples are full of fiber, antioxidants and vitamins, so they'll make you feel amazing.

Avocado—a plate of mashed avocado on homemade toast with lime juice, black pepper and chili is simple, but divine (page 42). Try it with my Superfood Bread. The recipe is in my first book. If you're sensitive to wheat but not to gluten, rye bread is a great option, too, and easy to find. And if you can't get either, rice cakes are great! Avocados are great in smoothies, as they make them creamy (pages 47–51). These green beauties are so good for you, too: anti-inflammatory, full of vitamins A,

C and E—important for beautiful skin and for strengthening the immune system—lots of fiber and amazing fats, to help you glow from the inside out.

Chia seed—a real super-food: tiny but powerful. I use them both for their nutritional content and their ability to thicken and bind mixtures. They're packed with a crazy amount of fiber, omega-3 fatty acids, protein, iron, calcium, magnesium, zinc and pretty much everything else you could ever need! This means they're great for digestive health, glowing skin, strong bones, high energy and balanced blood sugar.

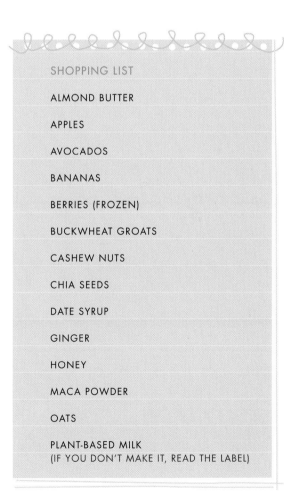

SHOPPING LIST

ALMOND BUTTER

APPLES

AVOCADOS

BANANAS

BERRIES (FROZEN)

BUCKWHEAT GROATS

CASHEW NUTS

CHIA SEEDS

DATE SYRUP

GINGER

HONEY

MACA POWDER

OATS

PLANT-BASED MILK
(IF YOU DON'T MAKE IT, READ THE LABEL)

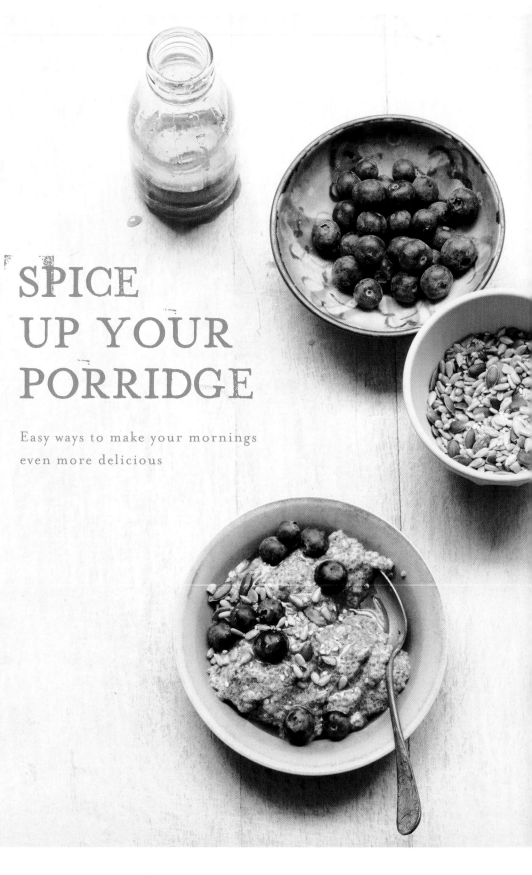

SPICE UP YOUR PORRIDGE

Easy ways to make your mornings
even more delicious

Chia pots are the easiest breakfast, and you can make two or three servings in one go and then store them in the fridge to enjoy in the morning. This pot has a thick, creamy texture with hints of rich coconut and almond butter, plus some warming cinnamon and ginger. I love it just as it is if I'm in a hurry, but if I have more time then I always top my bowl with banana slices, berries, seeds and granola to make it extra delicious.

MAPLE CHIA POTS

Serves 2

1¼ cups almond milk
2 heaping tablespoons
　　maple syrup
2 tablespoons almond butter
2 tablespoons shelled hemp seeds
2 teaspoons coconut oil
2 teaspoons ground cinnamon
2 teaspoons ground ginger
½ cup plus 2 tablespoons chia
　　seeds
berries and/or sunflower and
　　pumpkin seeds, to serve

Pour the milk into a bowl and stir in the maple syrup, almond butter, hemp seeds, coconut oil and spices. Mix everything well, until smooth.

Stir in the chia seeds.

Pour the mixture into a glass jar with a lid and leave in the fridge overnight, or for at least 6 hours, so that it sets and the chia seeds expand. This is fine kept in the jar in the fridge for up to 2 days. Return to room temperature to serve, with berries and seeds, if you like.

Kitchen Know-How

If your almond butter isn't very runny, then blend it with the milk first, before stirring in the chia seeds.

Nut-Free

If you don't eat nuts, then switch the almond butter to tahini.

If you're new to overnight oats, then I'd recommend you start with my classic Bircher Muesli (page 30), as it has a more conventional flavor, but once you're ready for something new, this is the recipe to choose. It's absolutely incredible, one of my favorite breakfasts ever. The taste is unique, while the puréed beets, apple and banana make each bite so creamy. It's also the most beautiful pink color, which always cheers up a weekday morning!

SWEET BEET OVERNIGHT OATS

Serves 2

1 small beet

1 apple

1 tablespoon maple syrup

1 tablespoon almond butter

1 banana

1¾ cups rolled oats

2 tablespoons shelled hemp
  seeds (optional)

2 tablespoons chia seeds

Preheat the oven to 425°F (convection 400°F), then place the beet in a baking pan and allow it to cook for 45 minutes to 1 hour, until the skin can easily be peeled off. (If you're using a pre-cooked beet, you can skip this step.)

Once the beet has cooled, peel the skin off with your fingers (discard it) and place the beet in a blender.

Peel and core the apple, chop it into a few pieces, then place these in the blender too.

Add a generous ¾ cup of water, the maple syrup, almond butter and banana to the blender and blend for 30 seconds or so, until the mixture is smooth.

Pour your oats into 2 jars (with lids), then pour half the blended mixture over each. Add half the hemp seeds and chia seeds to each jar and mix well.

Put the lids on the jars and place them in the fridge to soak overnight, or for at least 4 hours. This will keep in the jars for up to 2 days. Return to room temperature to serve.

Tweak It

This is also delicious served hot: simply place the soaked oats into a pan, add a little oat milk and allow to warm up for a minute or so, watching carefully that the pan doesn't get dry.

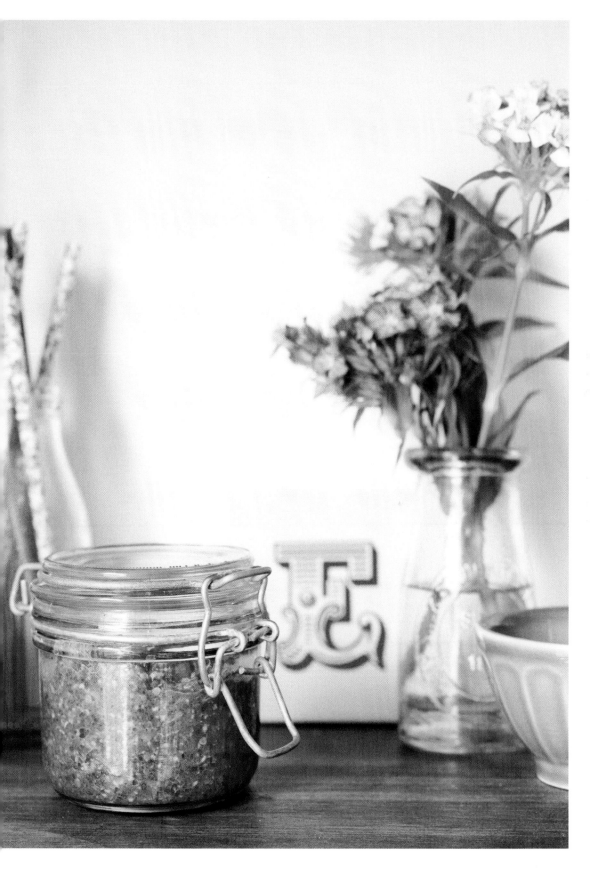

A great, useful breakfast if your mornings are rushed, as it's really portable and only takes a couple of minutes to throw together. I eat it during the summer instead of hot porridge; it tastes just as good but is more appealing when it's warm outside. I love serving it with fresh fruit and granola, for a little crunch.

RAW BUCKWHEAT BOWLS

Serves 2

1¼ cups buckwheat groats
1 ripe banana
big handful of blueberries (about
    4 ounces), plus more
    to serve (optional)
5 tablespoons plant-based milk
1 tablespoon almond butter
1 tablespoon chia seeds
1 tablespoon honey, date syrup
    or maple syrup (optional)
dried fruit and seeds,
    to serve (optional)

Place the buckwheat in a bowl and cover it with about 1¼ cups of water. Cover and let this sit overnight to soak.

Once you're ready to make your porridge, drain the water from the buckwheat and rinse it well; it will be a bit gooey, so keep rinsing until the water runs clear from the sieve.

Add two-thirds of the buckwheat to a blender with all the other ingredients. Blend the mixture for 30 seconds or so, until it is creamy but not totally smooth.

Pour into a bowl or glass and stir in the remaining one-third of the buckwheat before eating, with more blueberries and a sprinkling of dried fruit and seeds, if you like. This is fine kept in an airtight container in the fridge for up to 2 days. Return to room temperature to serve.

Tweak It

You can use any fruit in this, try replacing the blueberries with strawberries, raspberries or blackberries, or even substitute mango for the banana.

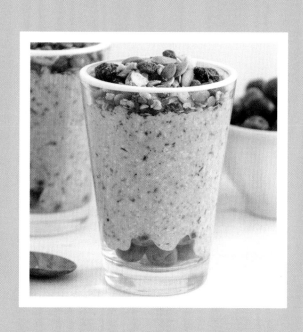

『BUCKWHEAT–
LOVELY LITTLE GRAINS
OF GOODNESS!

A lifesaver when you're busy! I normally make three servings at once and keep them in the fridge (just scale the recipe up to do the same), so that they're ready to go in the morning. I find that it's delicious just as it is thanks to the grated apple and raisins, but you can also add a little syrup or honey as suggested in the recipe if you like.

BIRCHER MUESLI

Serves 1

1 apple
generous ½ cup rolled oats
¼ cup raisins
5 teaspoons sunflower seeds
1 tablespoon chia seeds
generous ½ cup cashew milk (or
   any other plant-based milk)
1 teaspoon maple syrup, date
   syrup or honey (optional)
handful of blueberries,
   raspberries or strawberries
   (optional)

Grate the apple into a bowl, then add all the other ingredients and stir it all together.

Place the mixture into an airtight jar and leave in the fridge for about 6 hours to allow the oats to soften and absorb the milk. Then continue to store in the fridge for up to 3 days. Return to room temperature to serve.

Tweak It

If you want to make this extra creamy, add 1 tablespoon of coconut yogurt; it creates the most wonderful texture.

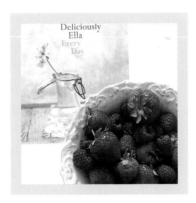

If you're not a fan of oats—or find that you're getting bored with traditional oatmeal—then this quinoa version will make you really happy! Using quinoa will give you great energy for the day, as it's full of plant-based protein. It also tastes delicious as each bite is bursting with hints of honey, banana and ginger.

QUINOA AND GINGER PORRIDGE

Serves 1

⅓ cup quinoa

½ cup plus 2 tablespoons plant-based milk

1 tablespoon honey

1 banana

½ teaspoon ground ginger

Place the quinoa in a saucepan with ⅔ cup of boiling water, the milk and honey and allow the mixture to come to a boil.

Once the porridge is boiling, reduce the heat and simmer for about 15 minutes, until the quinoa is fluffy and most of the liquid has been absorbed (you don't want it to be dry though).

About 5 minutes before the porridge is ready, slice the banana into the mixture and stir in the ginger, then let everything cook together for the remaining time before serving.

Tweak It

Try adding lots of nuts, seeds and raisins to this to make it extra delicious.

Porridge is my favorite breakfast and in winter I eat it almost every day. This is the best version for weekday mornings, as you soak the oats while you get dressed, so they only need to cook for a few minutes. All four flavors are delicious and I mix them up during the week for variety. I especially like the almond butter variation if I'm going to yoga or the gym in the morning, as it's full of energizing plant-based protein.

SPEEDY PORRIDGE, FOUR WAYS

All serve 1

ALMOND BUTTER AND HEMP

¾ cup rolled oats
scant ½ cup plant-based milk
I teaspoon coconut oil
I teaspoon honey or maple syrup (optional)
½ teaspoon ground ginger
2 tablespoons almond butter
shelled hemp seeds

Place the oats in a saucepan and pour in ½ cup plus 2 tablespoons of boiling water. Leave to soak for 10 minutes; all the water should have been absorbed and they should be just about soft enough to eat.

Pour in the milk, coconut oil (this adds flavor and texture), honey and ginger. Add half the almond butter.

Cook for 5–10 minutes, until it's nice and creamy and the oats are really soft.

Serve, with the remaining almond butter and a sprinkling of hemp seeds on top.

Kitchen Know-How

Be careful of different types of oats! Quick-cooking oats take only 3 or 4 minutes to cook; soaking turns them to mush. Extra-thick rolled oats take much longer and need more liquid. Use standard rolled oats instead.

BANANA AND HONEY

¾ cup rolled oats
scant ½ cup plant-based milk
I heaping teaspoon honey
I banana, sliced

Soak the oats and cook as before with half the banana. Serve with the remaining banana.

CINNAMON AND DATE

¾ cup rolled oats
scant ½ cup plant-based milk
4 medjool dates, pitted and chopped
I heaping teaspoon ground cinnamon
I teaspoon coconut oil

Soak the oats and cook as before.

RAISIN AND APPLE

¾ cup rolled oats
handful of raisins
scant ½ cup plant-based milk
I red apple, coarsely grated
½ teaspoon vanilla powder
I teaspoon maple syrup

Soak the oats with the raisins. Cook as before.

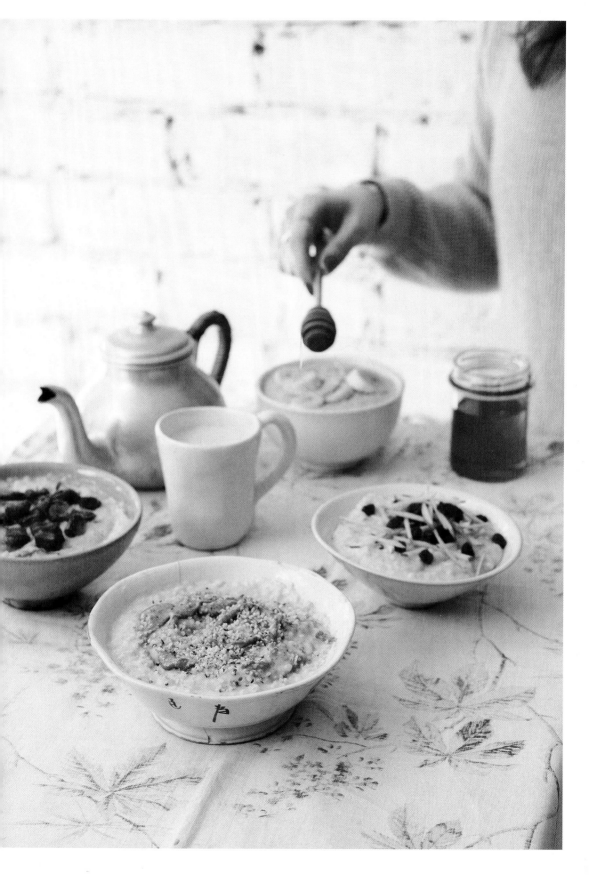

BAKED
DELICIOUSNESS

The sweet smell of breakfast

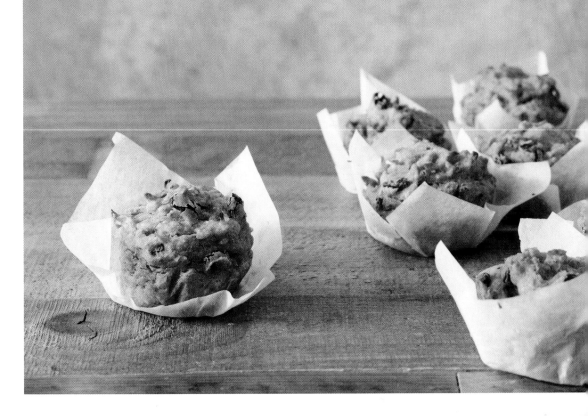

These are the best breakfasts if you like something super-portable to eat on the go. They make a great mid-morning or afternoon snack for the same reason. The wonderful thing is that they are predominantly sweetened with apple and carrot, with just a splash of maple syrup and honey, so they're not too sweet at all. I like spreading a little almond butter over my muffin, it's so good!

CARROT CAKE MUFFINS

Makes 12

2¾ cups grated carrots
¾ cup grated apples
¾ cup rolled oats
1 cup plus 1 tablespoon
    buckwheat flour
½ cup raisins
1 tablespoon chia seeds
1 tablespoon ground cinnamon
1½ tablespoons coconut oil
4 tablespoons Apple Purée
    (page 40)
3 tablespoons maple syrup
2 tablespoons honey
generous 1 cup almond milk

Preheat the oven to 325°F (convection 300°F).

Place the grated carrots and apples and all the dry ingredients together in a large bowl.

Melt the coconut oil in a small saucepan and add it to the bowl with all the other ingredients. Mix everything together well.

Line a 12-cup muffin tin with paper liners and scoop the mixture in.

Bake for 35 minutes, until the tops turn a golden brown.

Take them out of the oven and let them sit for 10 minutes to cool slightly in the tin and finish setting. Remove them from the tin and leave on a cooling rack for 20 more minutes.

Once completely cool, store in an airtight container at room temperature; they should last for about 5 days.

I think this might be the healthiest breakfast you could have, and it goes from fridge to plate in less than ten minutes. After a bowlful you'll feel like a superhero all day! Eating this for breakfast also means that, before you've even started your day, you've had four great portions of veggies, which is awesome. If I'm not especially hungry, I love eating this just as it is, but on hungry mornings or for busy days I add some bread (which is why I've put the recipe in this section) and, when I'm feeling like a total goddess, I add sauerkraut on the side for probiotic goodness!

THE PERFECT GARDEN FRY-UP

Serves 1

2 tablespoons olive oil
½ teaspoon cayenne pepper
1 teaspoon dried oregano
1 teaspoon dried thyme
2 garlic cloves, crushed
salt and pepper
6 cremini mushrooms, very
   finely sliced
10 cherry tomatoes (halved
   or quartered if large)
juice of 1 lemon
2 ounces spinach
½ avocado

Pour the olive oil into a frying pan and add the cayenne pepper, oregano, thyme, garlic, salt and black pepper. Let it heat and develop its fragrance for 2 minutes.

Add the mushrooms, tomatoes and half the lemon juice and let everything cook for about 3 minutes, at which point the veg should have softened.

Stir in the spinach and let it wilt for another minute or so.

Pile the vegetables from the pan onto a plate—or a piece of toast—and slice the avocado on top.

Drizzle the remaining lemon juice over the avocado and sprinkle with a little salt and pepper to serve.

Tweak It

Make this as a weekend brunch for all your friends and family. If they or you eat eggs, then enjoy some poached eggs with it. I do this at home and everyone loves it!

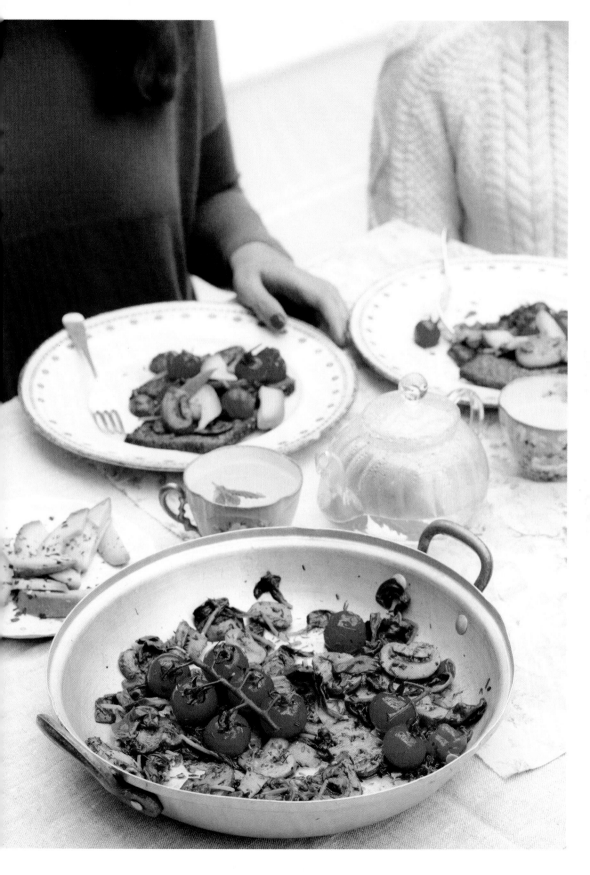

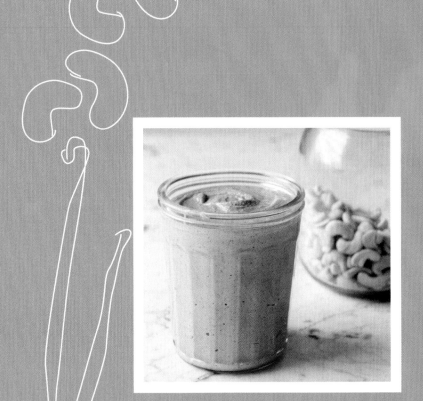

CASHEWS AND
VANILLA: MADE FOR
EACH OTHER

Honestly, this is outrageously good; it tastes and smells like cake mix! Last year I went through a phase when I was so obsessed with vanilla that I had to put it into absolutely everything I made, and this combination with cashews was my favorite. It's incredibly simple and just requires two ingredients, but it's one of the best tastes ever. You can spread it on toast, dip dates into it, drizzle it on porridge, blend it into smoothies, add it to banana ice cream . . . or just eat it straight from the jar!

CASHEW AND VANILLA BUTTER

Makes 1 large jar

14 ounces cashew nuts
2 teaspoons vanilla powder

Preheat the oven to 400°F (convection 350°F).

Spread the cashews on a baking sheet and cook for 10 minutes, or until they start to turn golden brown but aren't burnt. Leave to cool.

Place them in a powerful food processor with the vanilla powder and blend for about 10 minutes, until the mixture is totally smooth and creamy. It's so tempting to stop blending once it gets sticky, but keep going until it's runny; trust me, it's worth the extra few minutes! Stored in an airtight jar at room temperature, this will keep for a week or so.

Kitchen Know-How

Sadly, you do need a really strong processor, such as a Magimix, to make this successfully; a punier one won't render it totally smooth.

I love eating this with thick layers of almond butter and honey; it makes for the most delicious breakfast or snack. Baking this will make your kitchen smell totally divine, with wafts of vanilla and cinnamon swirling around. One of the things I love about this recipe is that it's not too sweet, which is why it's great for breakfast, as it is mainly sweetened by fruit—bananas and apples—with just a little maple syrup. I'm sure lots of you will be happy to hear that it is totally nut-free, too.

ZUCCHINI BANANA BREAD

Makes 1 loaf

2 tablespoons chia seeds
1 small zucchini (about
    4 ounces), coarsely grated
4 overripe bananas (1 pound,
    weighed in their skins),
    mashed, plus 1 more to
    decorate (optional)
1 vanilla pod, split, seeds
    scraped out
1¾ cups plus 2 tablespoons
    brown rice flour
¼ cup maple syrup
¼ cup Apple Purée (below right)
1 tablespoon ground cinnamon
coconut oil, for the pan

Preheat the oven to 400°F (convection 350°F).

Place the chia seeds in a mug with ½ cup of water. Set aside for 10 minutes, until the water has been absorbed and the chia has formed a gel; stir it halfway through so it's all absorbed evenly.

Put the zucchini into a bowl with the bananas and vanilla seeds. Mix in the flour, syrup, apple purée and cinnamon. Stir in the chia seeds and let everything sit for 10 minutes.

Oil a 9 x 5-inch loaf pan with coconut oil. Scoop the batter into the pan. Cut the last banana (if using) in half lengthwise and place it on top, gently pressing it in.

Bake for 45–50 minutes, then allow to cool. Stored in an airtight container, this lasts for 5 days.

Kitchen Know-How

Apple purée is super-simple. Peel and core 20 red apples. Chop into bite-size pieces. Place in a large saucepan with ¾ inch of water. Cook for 40 minutes, or until very soft, then blend until smooth. Add 3 tablespoons date or maple syrup, or 1 tablespoon ground cinnamon, or both. Store in the fridge for up to 5 days, or freeze in portions.

Make It Better

It's important that your bananas be really ripe for the texture and taste of this recipe, so it's worth waiting an extra few days to make this so that you can use brown bananas.

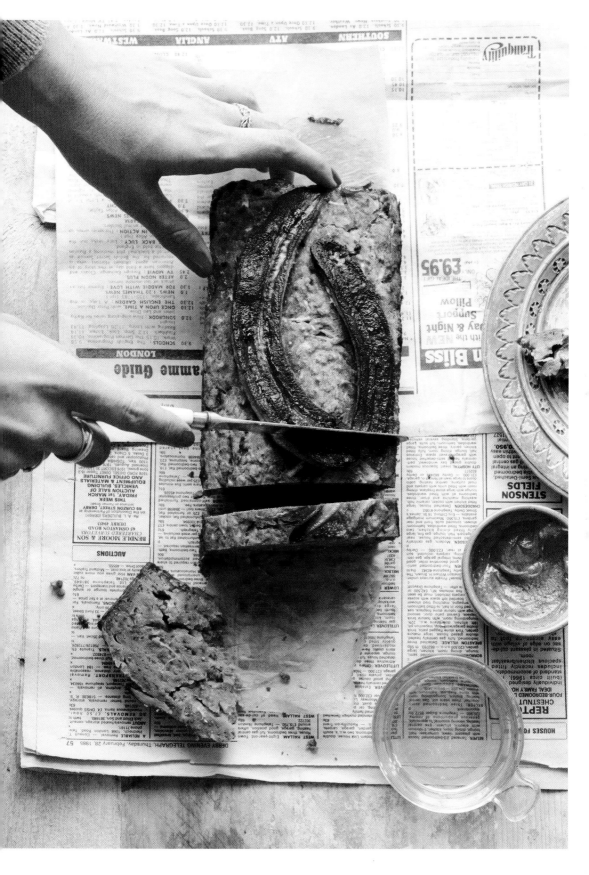

These two creations are my lazy breakfast saviors! I go for the chili-avocado option when I'm after something savory and the banana option when I need a little comfort in my life. Both take literally two minutes to throw together and, if you're really in a rush, you can even eat them as you walk out of the house.

TWO-MINUTE TOAST, TWO WAYS

Both serve 1

CHILI–AVOCADO

1 ripe avocado
juice of 1 lime
1 teaspoon olive oil
1 teaspoon chili flakes
salt and pepper
2 slices of toast

Scoop the avocado flesh out of the skin and place it in a shallow dish. Mash it with a fork until no lumps remain, then stir in the lime juice, olive oil, chili flakes, salt and lots of pepper.

Spread half over each piece of toast. Enjoy.

Make It Better

It's so important to use a soft, ripe avocado here, as otherwise the toast-topper will be lumpy rather than deliciously creamy! Likewise, you need a truly ripe banana for the sweet version, as this makes it so much sweeter, and will make mashing it far easier as it will be soft.

ALMOND BUTTER AND BANANA

1 ripe banana
1 tablespoon almond butter
2 slices of toast
sprinkling of sea salt

Slice the banana, then roughly mash it in a bowl with a fork. Mix in the almond butter.

Spread on the toast before sprinkling a little salt over it all.

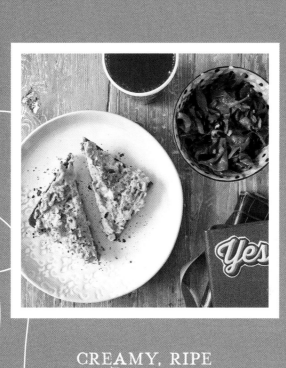

CREAMY, RIPE
AVOCADO SPIKED
WITH CHILI

The best grab-and-go breakfast! They're so much more delicious and nutritious than the bars you buy in a store, plus they're so easy to make. The mix of banana, cashew butter, honey, cinnamon and vanilla gives each bite a wonderfully moreish taste while the oats lend them a delicious, slightly chewy texture. If you love nut butter as much as I do, you might like spreading a layer of Cashew and Vanilla Butter (page 39) over the bar as you eat it; it's so good!

BANANA BREAKFAST BARS

Makes 10

2 very ripe bananas
2½ cups rolled oats
scant ½ cup almond milk
2 tablespoons cashew butter
I tablespoon ground cinnamon
I tablespoon honey
I teaspoon vanilla powder
coconut oil, for the dish

Preheat the oven to 350°F (convection 325°F).

Slice the bananas onto a plate and mash with a fork until smooth. Place in a bowl with all the remaining ingredients (except the coconut oil) and stir everything together.

Oil a baking dish or brownie pan (mine is 9 x 6 x 2 inches) with coconut oil and spoon the mixture into the dish.

Bake for about 12 minutes. Leave to cool, then cut into bars.

Store in an airtight container in the fridge for up to 5 days.

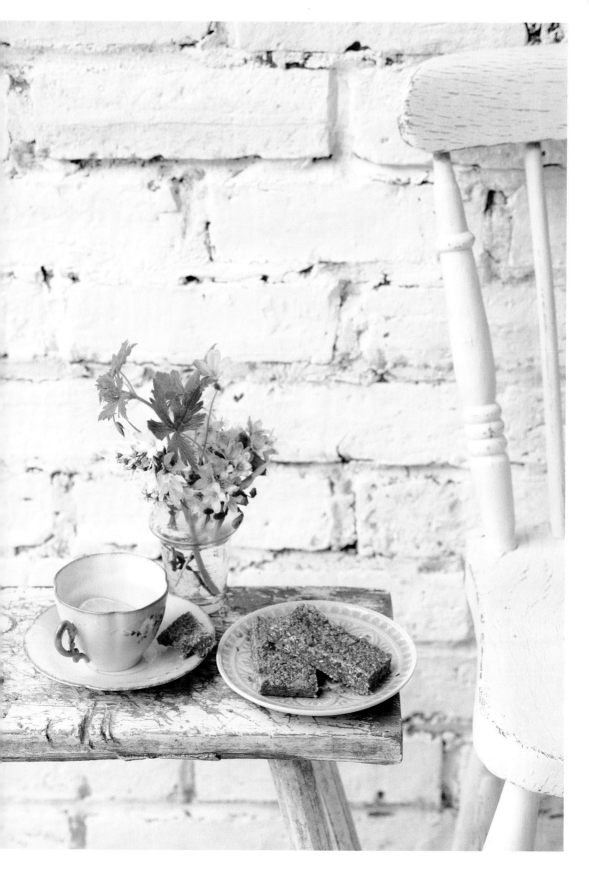

ENERGY-BOOSTING SMOOTHIES

Make friends with your blender

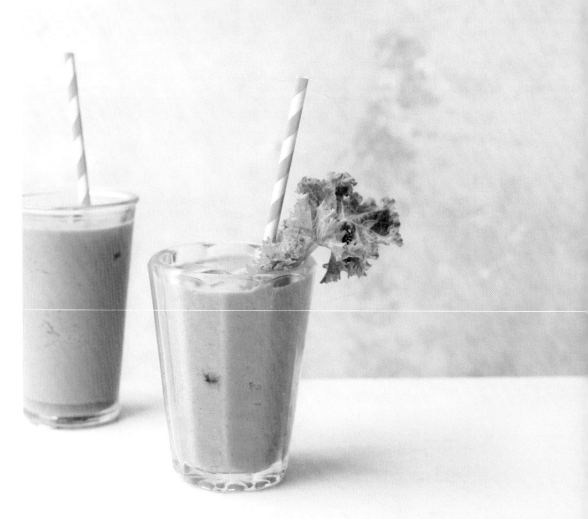

This is perfect for those days when you want lots of green goodness in your life. The banana and kale provide so many vitamins and minerals, while the nut butter and milk make it extra creamy. If you need a little more mellowness at breakfast time, add a little honey, but even if you don't, the fruit means you won't be holding your nose as you drink your veggies here!

A great breakfast or post-workout meal as it gives an incredible protein boost, especially from the cashew milk, hemp seeds and almond butter. All this protein plus the fiber in each of the ingredients does wonders for your energy level, so it will really get your day off to a happy start. Plus it literally takes two minutes to throw this together and requires no chopping at all!

KALE AND CUCUMBER SMOOTHIE

Serves 1

handful of kale
1 banana
¼ small cucumber, roughly chopped
handful of frozen berries
scant ½ cup plant-based milk
1 tablespoon nut butter

Tear the kale leaves from their stems and place them in a blender.

Add the banana to the blender with all the remaining ingredients. Blend until smooth.

Tweak It

If you don't like banana in this or any other smoothie, just leave it out and use a whole avocado, peeled and pitted, instead, along with 1 teaspoon of honey.

SUPER SPINACH SMOOTHIE

Serves 1

1 frozen sliced banana
generous ¾ cup cashew milk (page 53 for homemade, or use any other plant-based milk)
large handful of spinach
2 teaspoons shelled hemp seeds
1 teaspoon almond butter
1 teaspoon maca powder
1 medjool date, pitted

Simply place everything in a blender and blend until smooth.

Kitchen Know-How

Never freeze a banana whole; it will destroy your blender! Peel it, slice it and store the slices in the freezer in a freezer bag or airtight container.

This thick, creamy bowl is an awesome breakfast if you have a busy day ahead as it will give you so much energy. It's more filling than a smoothie and much thicker. It really feels like eating a big bowl of creamy yogurt, so it's perfect for those of you who are trying to move away from dairy but are missing your morning yogurt. I love topping my smoothie bowl with lots of berries, homemade granola and an extra dollop of almond butter for a delicious start to the day.

SWEET SMOOTHIE BOWL

Serves 1

6 strawberries

1 banana

½ avocado

5 tablespoons coconut milk, or other plant-based milk

1 tablespoon chia seeds

1 heaping tablespoon almond butter, plus more to serve (optional)

1 teaspoon maple syrup or honey (optional)

strawberries and mixed seeds, to serve (optional)

Cut the tops and any white core from the strawberries and place in a blender with the banana.

Scoop the avocado flesh out of the skin and add it to the blender with all the remaining ingredients, sweetening it with the maple syrup or honey if you want.

Blend until smooth. Serve with fruit and seeds sprinkled on top, if you like, or a drizzle of almond butter, or both.

Kitchen Know-How

If you're not planning on eating this within about 30 minutes of making it, then leave out the chia seeds, as otherwise it will set into more of a gelatin than a yogurt texture!

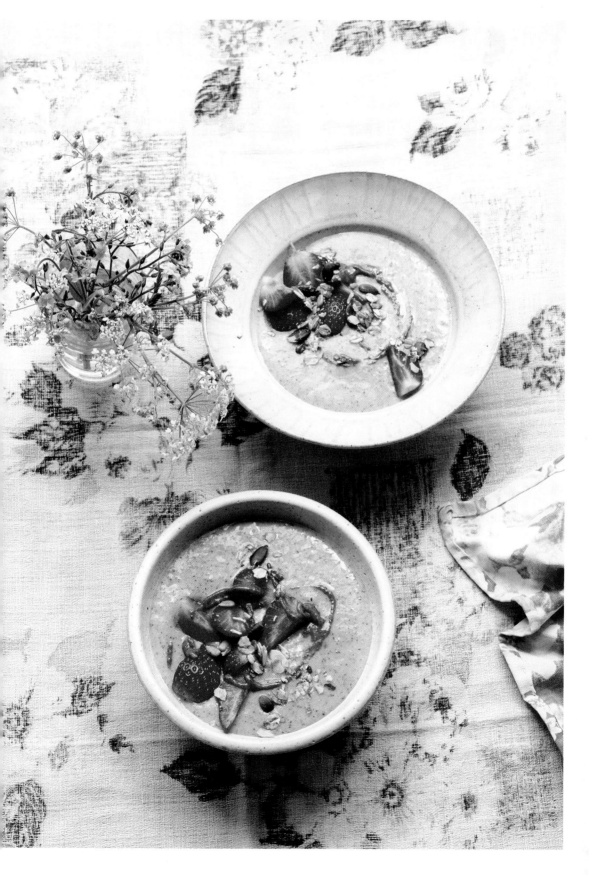

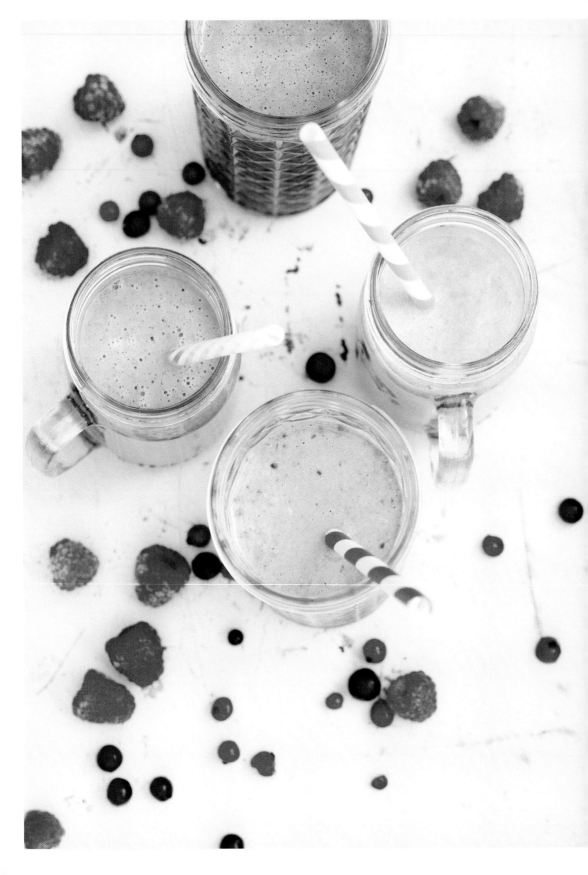

My go-to morning smoothies, these are so easy that I always keep the base ingredients—bananas, frozen berries and plant-based milk—in my kitchen and add other ingredients depending on what I feel like that morning. The mango and honey is the best if you need something soothing; the oat and cashew is perfect if you need lots of energy; spinach and almond butter is great for a protein boost; kale and cacao is ideal for a green kick!

MY MORNING SMOOTHIE, FOUR WAYS

All serve 1

For each one of these smoothies, just put all the ingredients in a powerful blender and blend until smooth. It may take a little longer to blend the oat mixture than the others, as the cashews need a little longer to break down.

KALE AND CACAO

small handful of kale, coarse ribs discarded
½ banana, peeled
½ avocado, peeled and pitted
1 teaspoon honey
1 tablespoon raw cacao powder
1¼ cups cashew milk (page 53 for homemade,
   or use any other plant-based milk)
1 teaspoon almond butter
a few ice cubes

Shop Sense

Buying packages of frozen berries is much cheaper than buying fresh berries and freezing them. You'll find them in most supermarkets and health food stores.

SPINACH AND ALMOND BUTTER

1 banana, peeled
handful of frozen berries
½ cup plus 2 tablespoons
   plant-based milk
big handful of spinach
1 tablespoon almond butter

MANGO AND HONEY

½ mango, peeled and pitted
handful of frozen berries
½ cup plus 2 tablespoons plant-based milk
1 banana, peeled
1 teaspoon honey

OAT AND CASHEW

1 banana, peeled
handful of frozen berries
½ cup plus 2 tablespoons
   plant-based milk
big handful of rolled oats
small handful of cashew nuts
1 teaspoon tahini

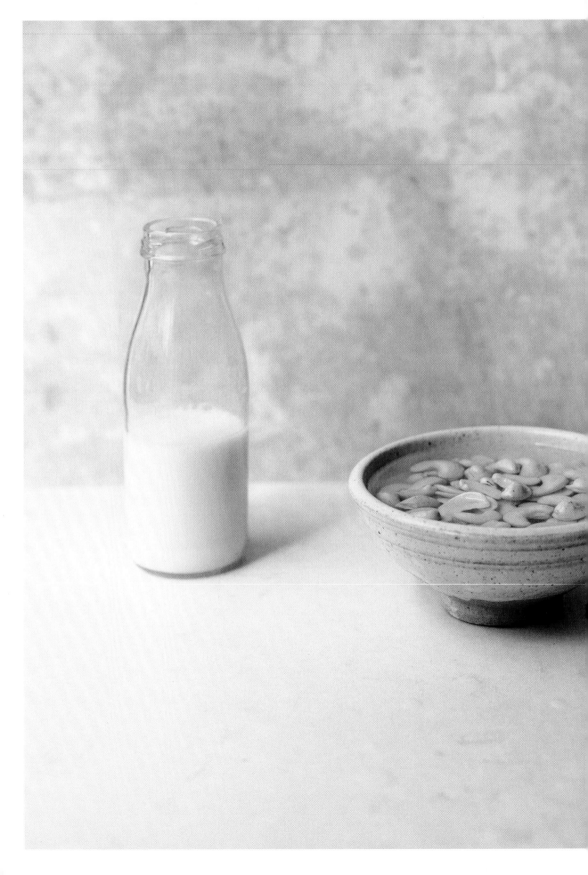

I have recently gone through a phase of making cashew milk all the time! It's been my favorite dairy-free milk by a long way, as it's so sweet and creamy. I use it in everything, especially at breakfast; it's amazing in porridge, smoothies and overnight oats.

CREAMY CASHEW MILK

Makes 1 quart

½ pound cashews

Simply soak the cashew nuts in a bowl of water overnight, or for at least 6 hours.

Drain the water and place the cashews in a powerful blender with 4 cups of fresh water. Blend for 1 minute or so until it looks smooth.

Pour the milk through a nut milk bag into a bowl, squeezing all the milk out of the bag as you go. Discard what's left in the bag and pour the milk into an airtight pitcher or sealable bottle.

Store in the fridge for up to 5 days.

Tweak It

Try adding a little honey or maple syrup to your cashew milk to make a sweet drink.

Kitchen Know-How

To make your own plant-based milks, you will need a nut milk bag to strain them through. These are widely available these days; just search online for "nut milk bag."

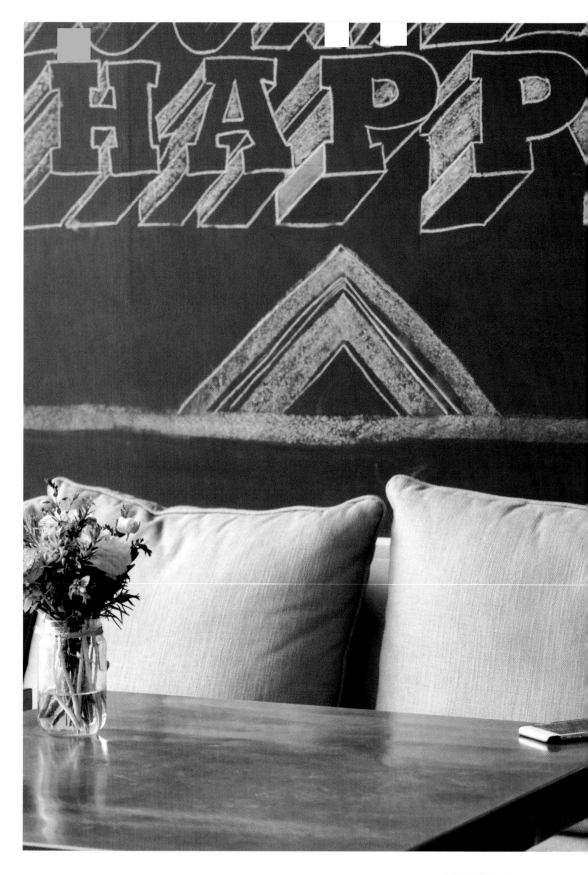

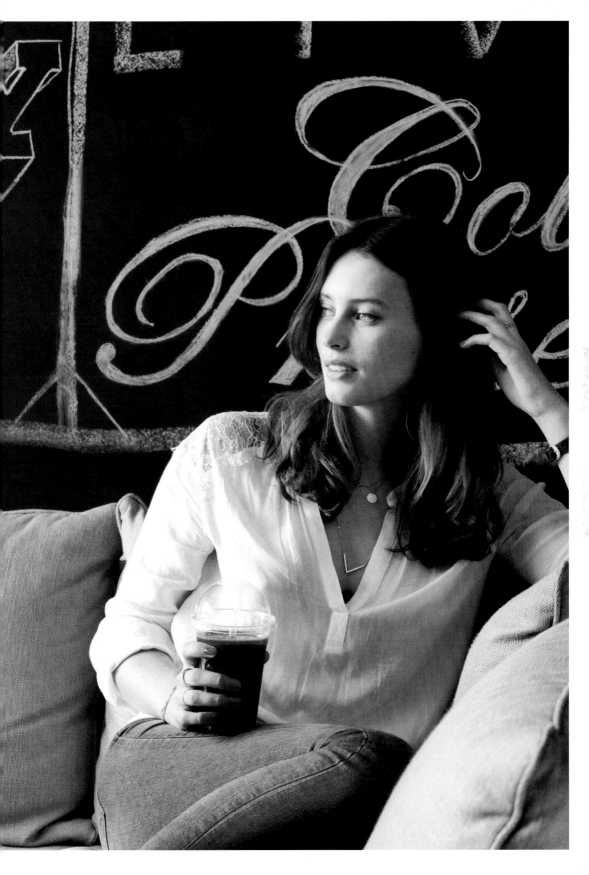

SWEET POTATO AND GARLIC PURÉE

SMOKY EGGPLANT DIP

BLACK BEAN HUMMUS

SPICY TURMERIC HUMMUS

FRESH MINT AND CASHEW PESTO

HEALTHY EATING
ON-THE-GO

MISO AND SESAME BROWN RICE

TAHINI BUCKWHEAT

LEMON QUINOA

SESAME MARINATED KALE

CASHEW COLESLAW

ZUCCHINI AND CARROT STRIP SALAD

SUN-DRIED TOMATO AND ZUCCHINI NOODLES

BAKED TOMATO CHICKPEAS

PERFECT PESTO VEGGIES

SPICED SQUASH AND SWEET POTATO CHUNKS

ROASTED PARSNIP "FRIES"

CARROT, BEET AND SESAME SALAD

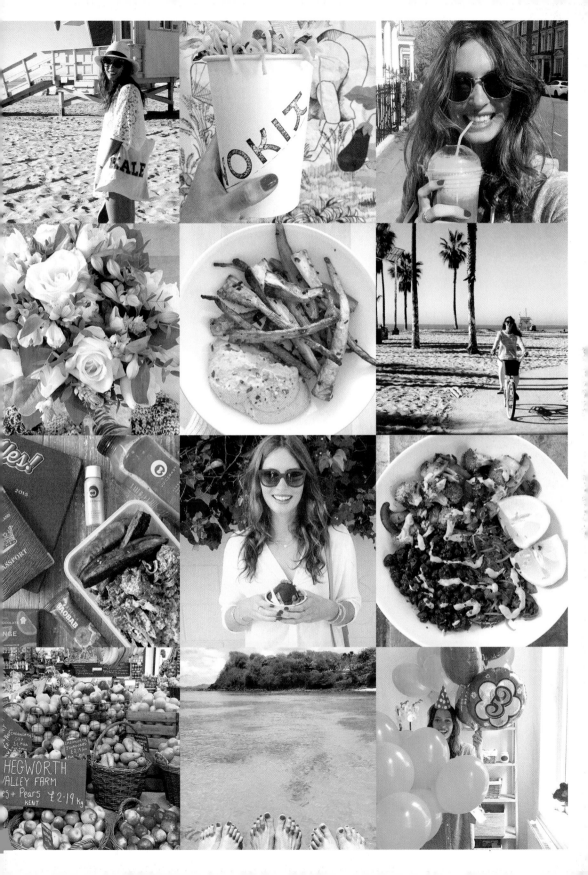

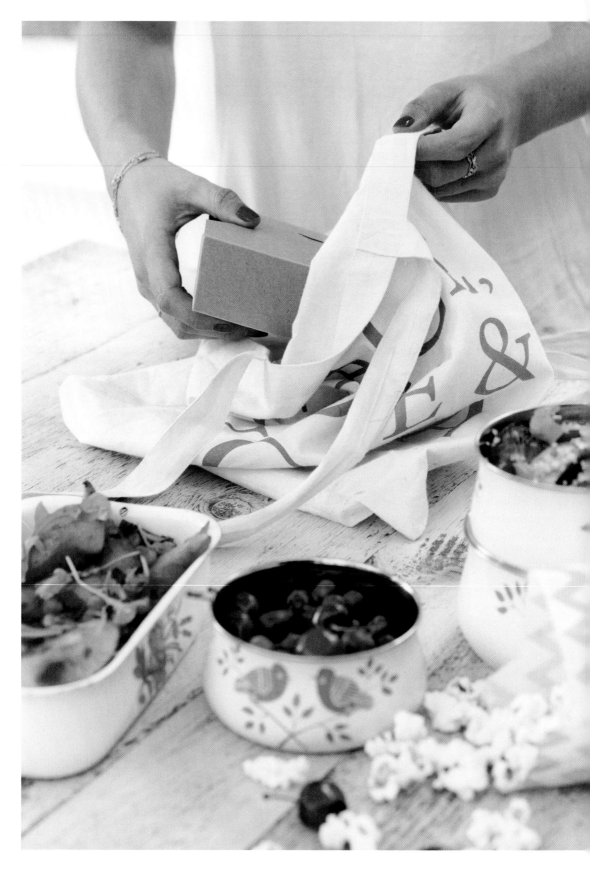

HEALTHY EATING ON-THE-GO

While the Western world is definitely becoming more and more interested in healthy eating, it can still be hard to find delicious, nutritious meals when you're out and about. More often than not your options are a sandwich or a plain salad, neither of which is especially appealing. If you're new to the Deliciously Ella way of eating and trying to avoid things such as gluten and dairy, you'll inevitably pick the unexciting salad—and I would do the same—but it's likely to leave you feeling uninspired and probably hungry. So, instead, I want to introduce you to some fantastic on-the-go options that will get you buzzing with energy and help you to fall in love with plant-based eating.

Staying healthy when you're really busy or out at work all day can be easy and very delicious. All it takes is a little bit of organization. I do understand that finding the time and energy to be this prepared may seem like an impossible task but, trust me, it's way more do-able than you might think and it makes the world of difference! I know that our lives don't go to plan one hundred percent of the time, but if you prepare well and have some easy things stashed in the fridge to grab when you're running late, or if plans change, then staying healthy and feeling awesome are going to be a lot more manageable. Plus, it's worth remembering that taking your own food with you normally tastes better, while also giving you more fuel to power through the day as each bite will nourish and support your body. It's normally less expensive to prepare your own meals, too, so you're really winning on all fronts here.

I love knowing that I have a box of rainbow goodness to be excited about. Before I got super-organized and starting doing this, I would get serious food envy when people around me starting eating their lunch while I chomped on the world's least exciting green salad. This was even harder when I first changed my diet and my taste buds still craved sugar rather than avocado and kale, as I found that whenever I left a meal unsatisfied, I started craving everything I was trying to avoid, notably cookies, cakes and chocolate! My palate has now changed and I no longer dream of processed sugar (yay!), but I do still find it difficult to leave a meal hungry and uninspired, so I really value the importance of being organized with my food.

So how do you fit it in? In short, you need to find a couple of hours twice a week to prepare delicious things. This may sound like a lot of time, but it's so worth it and it quickly becomes a habit. I always make my on-the-go food on Sunday and Wednesday evenings and it's become a little ritual! I'll hang out in my kitchen, dance around to some music and get creative until I've filled lots of airtight boxes with exciting dishes, which will form the basis of my lunches for the next few days. In fact, it's a great way to switch off from the world and have some me-time. Try not to see it as a chore, instead view it as a chance to explore new recipes and relax. Maybe persuade a family member or a friend to join you in the kitchen, so you can catch up and cook at the same time, or, if you're not a fan of cooking, then watch your favorite TV show as you chop: just find a way to make it fun.

No matter how busy your life is, I promise that you really do have two hours or so twice a week to cook foods that will make you look and feel your best. It may mean that you have to reschedule something else to prioritize your health, but investing in wellness is really the best commitment you can make.

Every week I find that I'm so grateful to myself for making that time, even if I didn't really want to. I love that I can take just two minutes in the morning to grab a delicious rainbow bowl filled with Spicy Turmeric Hummus, Miso and Sesame Brown Rice, Sesame Marinated Kale (pages 66, 71 and 75) and roast veggies; it makes me so happy. It means I can run around all day without getting exhausted or worrying that I won't find anything good or nourishing to eat, plus I get pretty grumpy when I'm hungry so it's always good to avoid that!

I base my on-the-go meals on three categories—dips and spreads, grains and veggies—this keeps it as simple as possible, which saves you precious prep time. I then combine the three elements in one container, so I have a delicious, varied meal to take with me. Each time I cook food I pick one dip, one grain and a couple of veggie dishes— then make portions of each to store in the fridge, so I can have a little every day. Of course, eating the same thing all week would get boring, so I also buy a variety of other veggies that I add to my lunch as I assemble it in the morning. For this, I focus on things that won't take more than a minute or two to prepare. I love using cherry tomatoes, arugula, avocados, olives, pomegranate seeds, spinach, artichoke hearts, pumpkin and sunflower seeds, raisins, sun-dried tomatoes and pine nuts. I'll buy three or four of that selection each week, so I can keep things interesting, then I finish my lunch box off by drizzling lots of lovely extra virgin olive

oil and lemon juice over everything. And don't forget that my great soups also make an excellent portable meal (pages 127–134).

For my dips and spreads I love using things such as hummus, Smoky Eggplant Dip, creamy Sweet Potato and Garlic Purée and Fresh Mint and Cashew Pesto (pages 65 and 68). I find they each add really nice textures, while also bringing all the different elements of the meal together, sort of in the same way as a dressing.

For my grains I use brown rice, quinoa or buckwheat groats. I cook them all in slightly different ways to keep them interesting, although you can mix and match the flavor combinations with the different grains, as they all work well together. I normally add sesame oil and miso to rice, lemon to quinoa and creamy tahini to buckwheat; this way all the grains have so much flavor, which helps bring your lunch to life. My veggie dishes vary hugely from a raw Cashew Coleslaw to Baked Tomato Chickpeas; classic roast veggies with tomato pesto to Roasted Parsnip "Fries" (pages 78, 83, 84 and 87), all of which are truly amazing.

I also find packed lunches a real lifesaver when I travel. Traveling can be really tricky for those of us who love eating well, as we all know that airports and train stations are practically the antithesis of health food shops! So I always travel with lots of my own food. The important thing to note here is that you'll have to forgo your dip, smoothie or spread if you're going through an airport; sadly, they count as a liquid and security will take your meal away from you. You can, however, take any solid food. Flight attendants think I am totally crazy as I take out my various boxes and decline their meals, but it means that I arrive at the destination feeling awesome and energized rather than sleepy and bloated, and that my trip is off to a much better start! I always take snacks with me, too, if it is a long flight. I normally also take sweet things, such as my Cinnamon and Honey Energy Bites and a bag of sweet Trail Mix (both in the Simple Sweets chapter, pages 204 and 208), as both travel really well and are great pick-me-ups.

When I go away for a few days I also take a travel blender with me; again I know this may sound a bit crazy but, honestly, it's a lifesaver. I find that if I have a smoothie every morning for breakfast I don't have to stress about whether I'm getting enough vitamins and minerals during the rest of my day and I continue to feel healthy and amazing throughout the trip.

When I arrive at my destination I go out and buy nuts, spinach, bananas and berries from a local market or supermarket and then blend them up every morning for an awesome breakfast. If I'm going away for more than a few days, I'll also take a couple of boosters with me so that I can make even better smoothies: my go-tos are chia seeds, hemp seeds, bee pollen and spirulina, as together these give you an incredible amount of protein, omega-3 fatty acids, iron and a whole heap of other vitamins and minerals that strengthen your body and your immune system.

MY TRAVEL CHECKLIST

A travel blender

Core smoothie ingredients: chia seeds, hemp seeds, bee pollen and spirulina

Homemade trail mix or energy balls, or any store-bought healthy snacks that can be carried in your bag, such as seeds, snack bars or crackers

A packed lunch for the travel day, plus a packed breakfast if you're leaving early; I find that Sweet Beet Overnight Oats or Bircher Muesli are the easiest to travel with (pages 26 and 30)

A glass water bottle (so you can refill it on the plane if you need to)

MY BUSY DAY CHECKLIST

A packed lunch using recipes in this chapter

Some snacks from the Simple Sweets chapter: Gooey Black Bean Brownies are great, as are Cacao, Oat and Raisin Cookies (pages 201 and 205)

A glass water bottle to make sure I stay hydrated all day

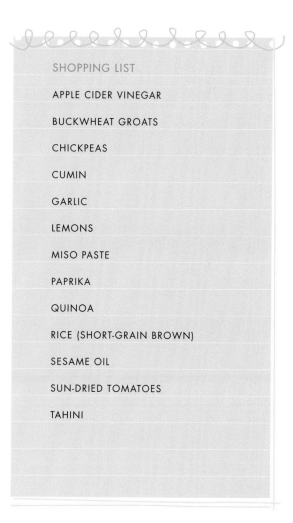

SHOPPING LIST

APPLE CIDER VINEGAR

BUCKWHEAT GROATS

CHICKPEAS

CUMIN

GARLIC

LEMONS

MISO PASTE

PAPRIKA

QUINOA

RICE (SHORT-GRAIN BROWN)

SESAME OIL

SUN-DRIED TOMATOES

TAHINI

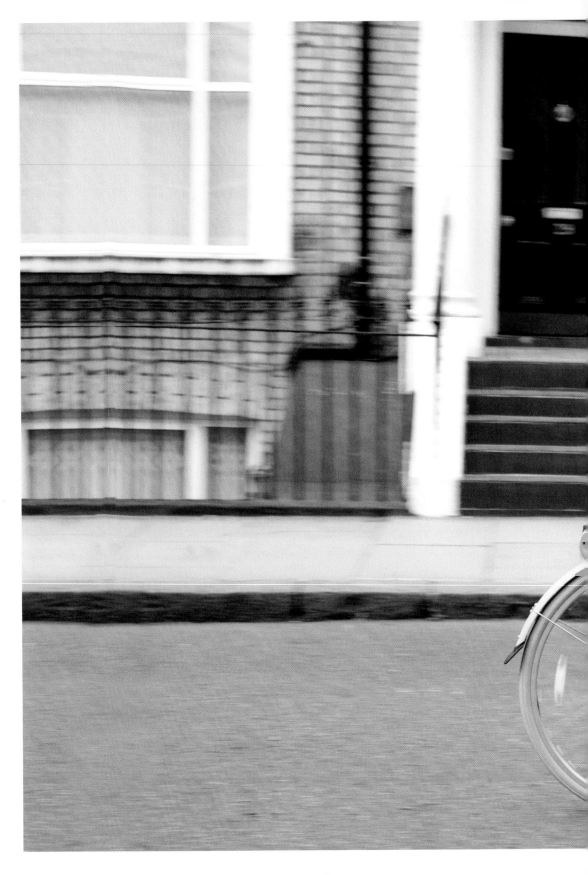

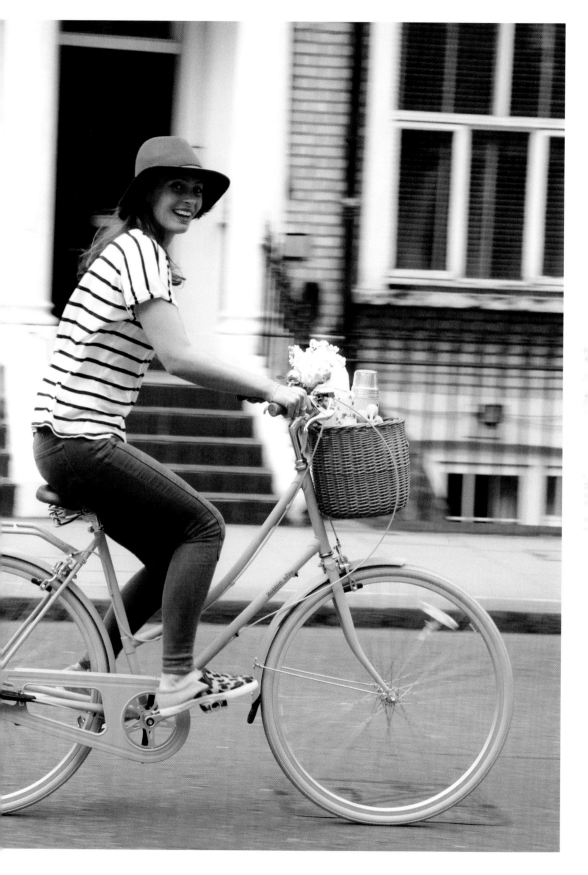

DELICIOUS DIPS

Creamy bowls of goodness to spice
up your lunch

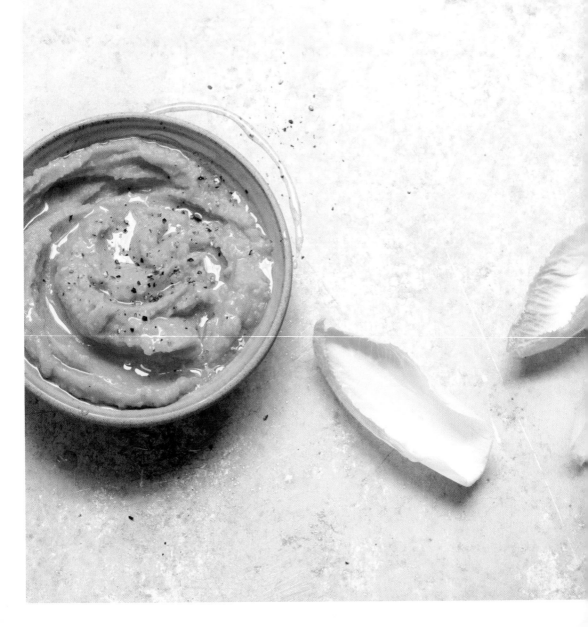

This is absolute heaven; I can't get enough of it. It goes with absolutely everything and instantly livens up any meal, plus it's so easy to make and only requires four simple ingredients. It's delicious served with my Honey and Mushroom Quinoa (page 150); the two go so perfectly together! It's great in a lunch box, too, as it adds a creamy texture and vibrant color to your meal, while also providing a wonderfully subtle sweetness.

SWEET POTATO AND GARLIC PURÉE

Makes 1 big bowl

3 sweet potatoes (2 pounds)
2 garlic cloves, crushed
juice of 1 lemon
salt
up to ½ cup plus 2 tablespoons
   almond milk

Peel the sweet potatoes and chop into small pieces. Place them in a steamer and steam for about 40 minutes, until each piece is so soft that it can easily be mashed by a fork. (If you don't have a steamer, you can also boil the sweet potatoes.)

Put the sweet potatoes in a food processor with the garlic, lemon juice and salt. Blend together, adding the milk bit by bit (you may not need it all), until totally smooth.

Remove the purée from the processer and leave it to cool. Store in an airtight container in the fridge for up to a week.

An old favorite of mine. This is one of the first dishes I made when I started learning to cook like this and I keep coming back to it. It's a wonderfully simple recipe and it keeps really well, plus it tastes equally awesome hot or cold, so it works all year round. In the summer it's a great snack with carrot sticks, while in the winter it's delicious really hot and mixed with a big bowl of quinoa and roasted veggies.

SMOKY EGGPLANT DIP

Makes 1 big bowl

4 eggplants
3 tablespoons tahini
9 ounces drained oil-packed
   sun-dried tomatoes
3 tablespoons apple cider vinegar
2 tablespoons tomato paste
2 tablespoons olive oil
juice of 1 lime
2 teaspoons ground cumin

Preheat the oven to 400°F (convection 350°F). Place the eggplants on a baking sheet and pierce with a knife; this is important, or they'll explode! Bake for 50 minutes, until tender and starting to look shriveled. Cool for a few minutes, then slice off the green tops and place in a food processor with the remaining ingredients.

Blend together until smooth, then store in an airtight container in the fridge for up to a week.

Kitchen Know-How

Let the eggplants cook for as long as possible, this gives a smoky flavor and creamy texture. It's better to overcook than undercook here!

I have a real hummus obsession, to the extent that I can't really go a day without it! As I eat it so often, I like to switch up the varieties, and this new black bean version has been my favorite for the last few months. I find it's much richer in flavor than the classic chickpea hummus (which I love), plus it normally comes out creamier, which is another bonus. I eat this in big salad bowls and with crackers or crudités for an afternoon snack. Try keeping a big bowl of this in your fridge to enjoy as an afternoon pick-me-up or post-workout snack, it's great at boosting energy.

I actually made this by accident. A friend and I were making the falafels from my first book and she misread the instructions: instead of pulse-blitzing the ingredients quickly into crumbs, she blended them into a dip. This was the best mistake ever as it created my all-time favorite hummus . . . which is a big statement from a hummus addict. I eat this almost every day with almost every dish; it's pretty addictive and instantly improves any meal. Make big batches to snack on any time, it's such a good livener. I love it with rice crackers, crudités . . . or just on a spoon!

BLACK BEAN HUMMUS

Makes 1 bowl

two 15-ounce cans black beans,
   drained and rinsed
scant ½ cup olive oil
1 tablespoon apple cider vinegar
juice of 1 lemon
2 tablespoons tahini
3 garlic cloves, crushed
2 teaspoons ground cumin
1 teaspoon ground coriander
½–1 teaspoon cayenne pepper
salt and pepper

Place everything into a food processor, pour in a scant 2 tablespoons of water and blend until smooth and creamy. Store in an airtight container in the fridge for up to a week.

SPICY TURMERIC HUMMUS

Makes 1 bowl

two 15-ounce cans chickpeas,
   drained and rinsed
½ cup plus 2 tablespoons olive oil
1 tablespoon date syrup
juice of 2 lemons
2 tablespoons apple cider vinegar
2 heaping tablespoons tahini
3 garlic cloves, crushed
2 teaspoons ground cumin
2 teaspoons ground coriander
2 teaspoons ground turmeric
1–2 teaspoons chili powder (depending
   how spicy you like it)
2 teaspoons paprika
salt and pepper

Place everything into a food processor, add 3 tablespoons of water and blend until smooth. Store in an airtight container in the fridge for up to a week.

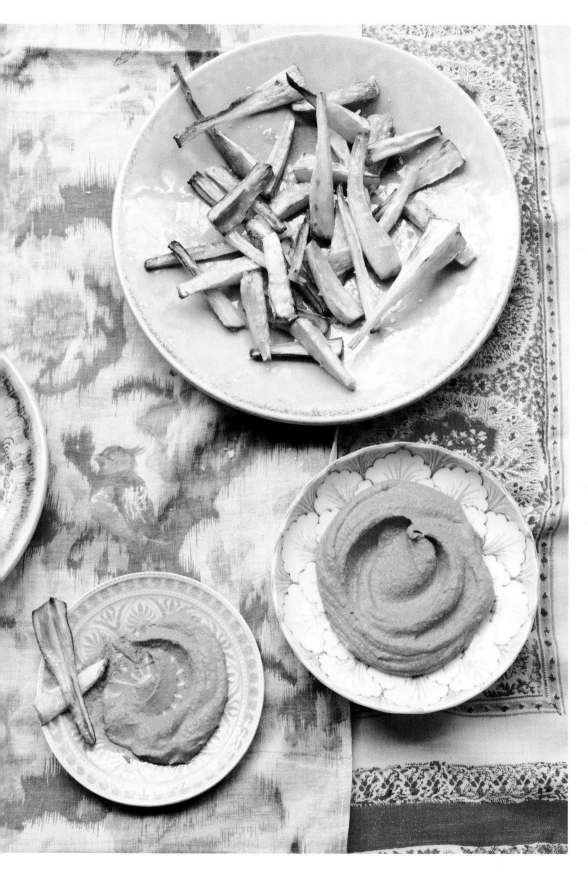

I love pesto; it instantly adds flavor to a meal and works as a great dressing, too. I use it in lunch boxes as a dressing to bring different elements together in one delicious bite. The mint flavor is quite subtle here, I didn't want it to be overpowering; instead it just adds a little freshness to your plate. This subtlety also means that the pesto works with just about everything. I especially love this with my Baked Tomato Chickpeas and Spiced Squash and Sweet Potato Chunks (pages 83 and 86), but it's amazing on its own, too, as a dip.

FRESH MINT AND CASHEW PESTO

Makes 1 bowl

1-ounce bunch of fresh mint
scant ½ cup olive oil, plus
   more to store
4 ounces pine nuts
2 ounces cashews
2 garlic cloves, crushed
juice of 1 lemon
salt

Tear the mint leaves from their stems.

Place all the ingredients into a food processor and blend for 30 seconds or so, to make a paste. Store in an airtight jar, making sure there is always a layer of olive oil on top to act as a seal. Keep in the fridge for up to a week.

Nut-Free

If you're allergic to nuts (or just don't like cashews much), use another 2 ounces of pine nuts instead of the cashews, it will still be lovely. Pine nuts are actually seeds, despite their name, so tend to cause fewer problems.

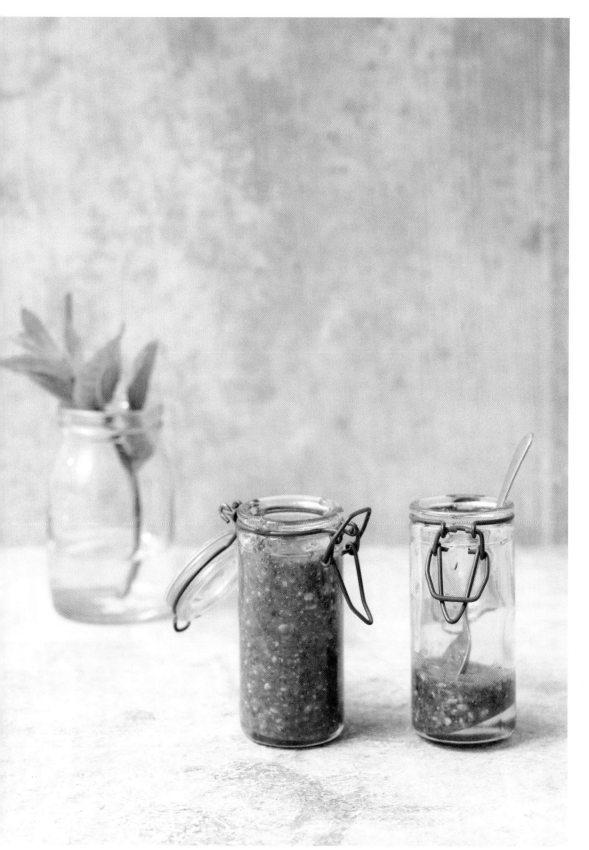

SIMPLE GRAINS

Tasty staples to boost your energy
and help you feel great

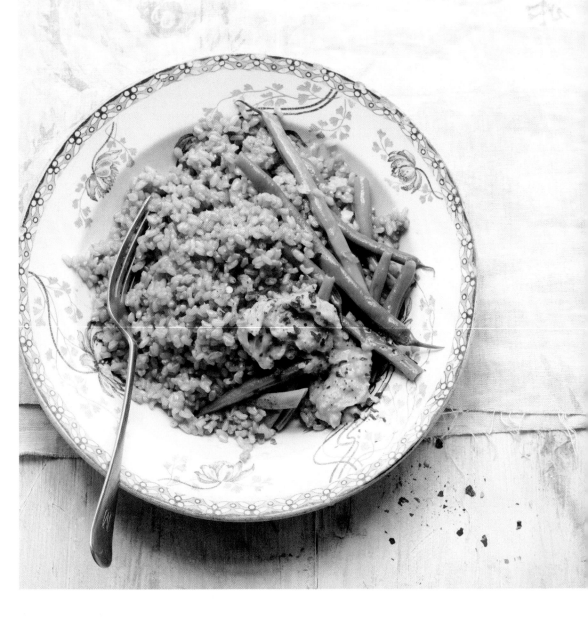

A staple in my house. I make it for my on-the-go lunches and to accompany any of my curry or stew dishes, as it tastes a million times more delicious than plain rice. The mix of tamari, sesame and miso paste gives it such a rich, deep flavor that works so well with almost everything, even simply with mashed avocado and sautéed garlicky green beans.

MISO AND SESAME BROWN RICE

Serves 3

1½ cups short-grain
  brown rice
1 tablespoon tamari
salt
1 tablespoon sesame oil
2 tablespoons olive oil
2 teaspoons miso paste

Place the rice into a saucepan with 3 cups of boiling water, the tamari and a sprinkling of salt. Bring to a boil, then reduce the heat to a simmer and place the lid on the pan. It should take about 45 minutes for the rice to cook, at which point all the water should have been absorbed.

Stir in the sesame oil, olive oil and miso paste and serve. If you're not eating it straight away, wait for it to cool down before placing it into an airtight container in the fridge.

Kitchen Know-How

If the cooked rice is a day or so old and looking a little sticky, drizzle olive oil over it: this will instantly revive it! And, when reheating cold rice, remember that you need to do so until every grain is steaming hot, for safety. Eat up any leftover rice within a couple of days.

This is the nuttiest, most flavorsome of the three grains I eat most, which is why I love it. The texture is denser than that of quinoa, but it feels lighter than brown rice. The tahini and olive oil mix make it wonderfully creamy, while the tamari adds a little salt; so together you get some pretty incredible works as the best base for any lunch on the road.

This is a real go-to for me. I like having it in my house at all times so that I can just throw it into any meal. It works so well with every veggie and it makes me feel so good. It's lighter than rice and buckwheat, so it's a great addition to an energizing lunch. I think it's especially good with Spicy Turmeric Hummus (page 66) and some roasted Spiced Squash and Sweet Potato Chunks (page 86).

TAHINI BUCKWHEAT

Serves 3

⅓ cup buckwheat groats
2 teaspoons tamari
salt
1 teaspoon olive oil
1 teaspoon tahini

Place the buckwheat into a saucepan with 1 cup plus 2 tablespoons of water, 1 teaspoon of the tamari and a little salt. Cook for 10 minutes, or until all the water has been absorbed and the buckwheat is cooked.

Stir in the second teaspoon of tamari, the olive oil and tahini.

Allow it to cool, before storing in an airtight container in the fridge. It will keep for up to 3 days.

LEMON QUINOA

Serves 3

generous 1 cup quinoa
juice of 1½ lemons
salt

Place the quinoa in a saucepan with the lemon juice and a little salt and pour in 2½ cups of water.

Bring to a boil over medium heat, then reduce the heat to a simmer and cook for about 15 minutes, until all the water has been absorbed.

Allow the quinoa to cool before placing it in an airtight container in the fridge. It will keep for up to 3 days.

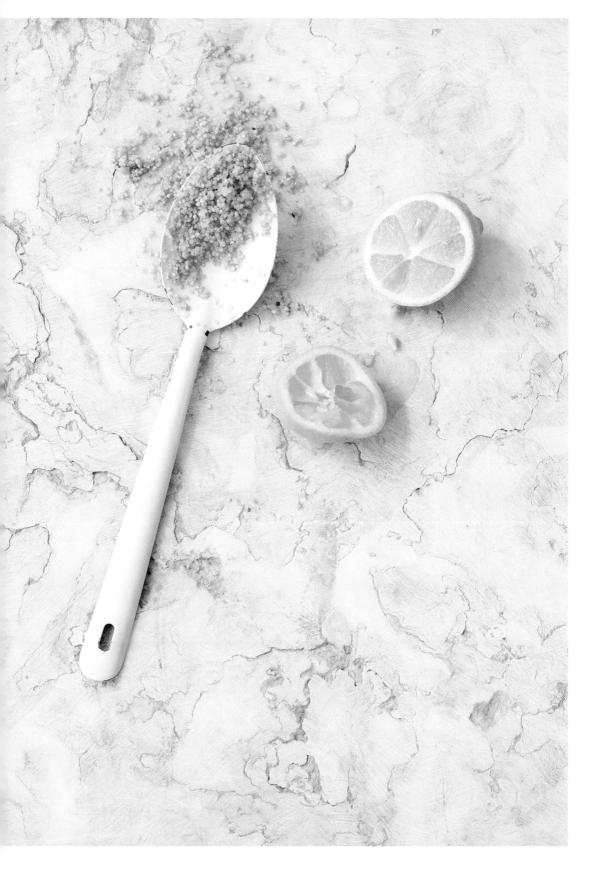

RAINBOW VEGGIES

Greens (and reds and oranges) on-the-go

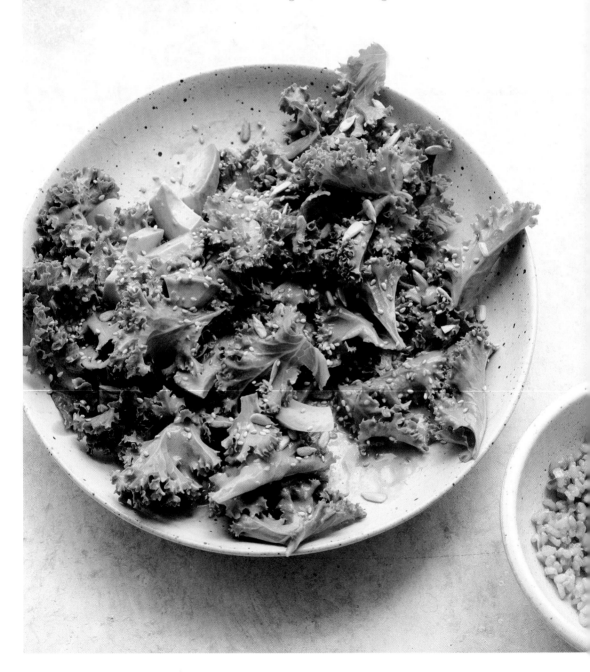

I've been living off marinated kale salads for the last few years; they're so easy to make and taste delicious with everything. This version is such a winner, too; the addition of sesame oil and sesame seeds is magical, it adds the most incredible flavor. The first time I tried this recipe I ate it almost every day for about a month. It's truly addictive.

SESAME MARINATED KALE

Serves 1

4 ounces kale
1½ tablespoons sesame oil
1 tablespoon apple cider vinegar
1 tablespoon olive oil
1 tablespoon tahini
1 teaspoon tamari
juice of ½ lime
handful of sesame seeds
handful of sunflower seeds

Tear the kale leaves from the stems and place the leaves in a bowl (discard the stems).

Pour the sesame oil, vinegar, olive oil, tahini, tamari and lime juice over the kale and firmly massage everything into the leaves for 1 minute or so, until they wilt and soften.

Use scissors to chop the leaves into really small pieces.

Sprinkle the sesame seeds and sunflower seeds over the salad to serve.

Make It Better

To make this salad heartier, try adding roasted veggies: beet, sweet potato, squash and potato are all great additions. Or add chunks of avocado, as we did for this photo. I also love pouring soup over this for a warming bowl of kale-spiked goodness.

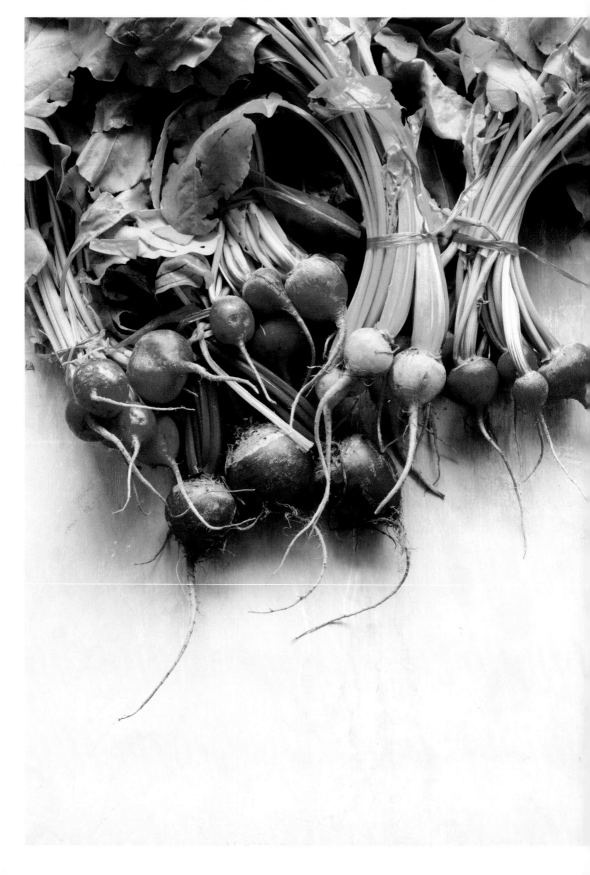

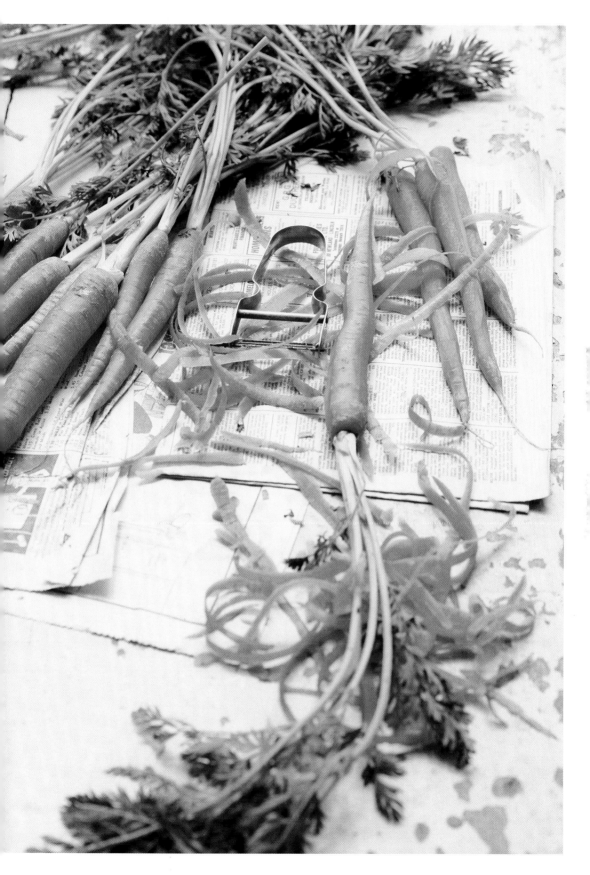

I used to hate coleslaw, but my mom kept asking me to make her a healthy version, so I played around with traditional recipes until I created this . . . which, it turns out, I absolutely love! It has such a creamy texture from the cashew-based dressing, which also adds so much flavor to each bite. It tastes pretty amazing with everything, especially bowls of grains with veggies.

CASHEW COLESLAW

Makes 1 big bowl

4 ounces cashews
scant ½ cup olive oil
1 tablespoon maple syrup
1 tablespoon tahini
juice of 1 lemon
1 garlic clove, crushed
2 carrots, coarsely grated
½ red cabbage, shredded

Place the cashews in a bowl, cover them with water and let them soak for at least 4 hours.

Drain the cashews and add them to a blender with all the other ingredients except the carrots and cabbage. Pour in a scant ½ cup of water and blend for 1 minute or so until a smooth, creamy mixture forms.

Stir the cabbage, carrots and dressing together in a bowl.

Nut-Free

If you can't eat nuts, then try switching the cashews for tofu and use a little less liquid in the dressing.

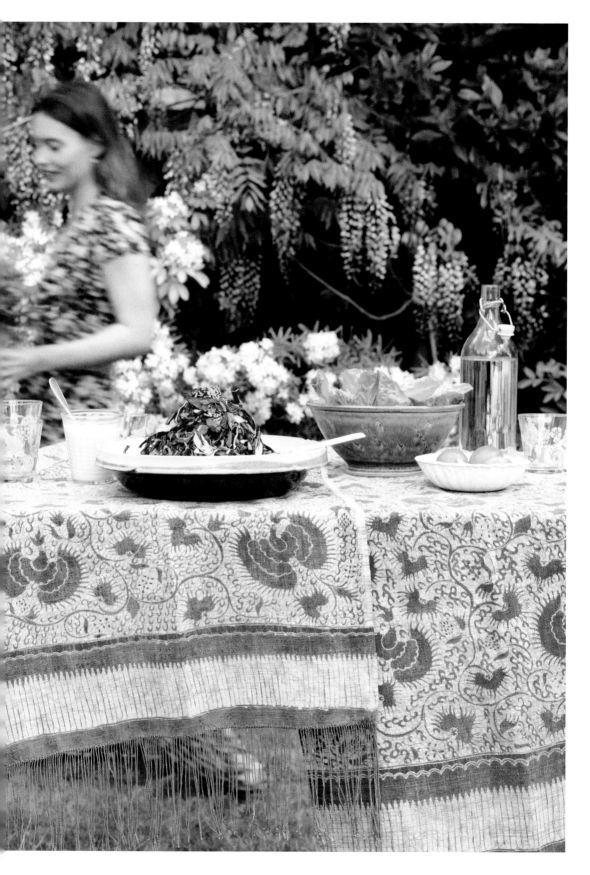

The easiest salad to box up and take with you. I love using the
zucchini and carrot strips as an alternative to leaves, I find they make
a great change to the usual salad base of lettuce, kale, arugula and so
on, adding so much more flavor as well as a chunkier, more interesting
texture. The mix of sunflower and pumpkin seeds adds a great crunch
to each bite, too, while the vinegar- and paprika-infused dressing
makes it all wonderfully rich and tangy.

ZUCCHINI AND CARROT STRIP SALAD

Serves 3

2 zucchini
3 large carrots
handful of pumpkin seeds
handful of sunflower seeds
¼ cup olive oil
2 tablespoons apple cider vinegar
I teaspoon paprika
salt and pepper

Use a vegetable peeler to peel the zucchini and carrots into
strips (peel and discard the outer layer of the carrots first).
I find it's hard to peel the very center of each veggie, so feel
free to discard (or nibble) this so that you don't end up
peeling your fingers!

Place the strips of carrot and zucchini in a bowl with the
seeds, pour the olive oil and vinegar over them, then
sprinkle the paprika, salt and pepper on top. Stir everything
well. It will keep, covered, in the fridge for up to 3 days.

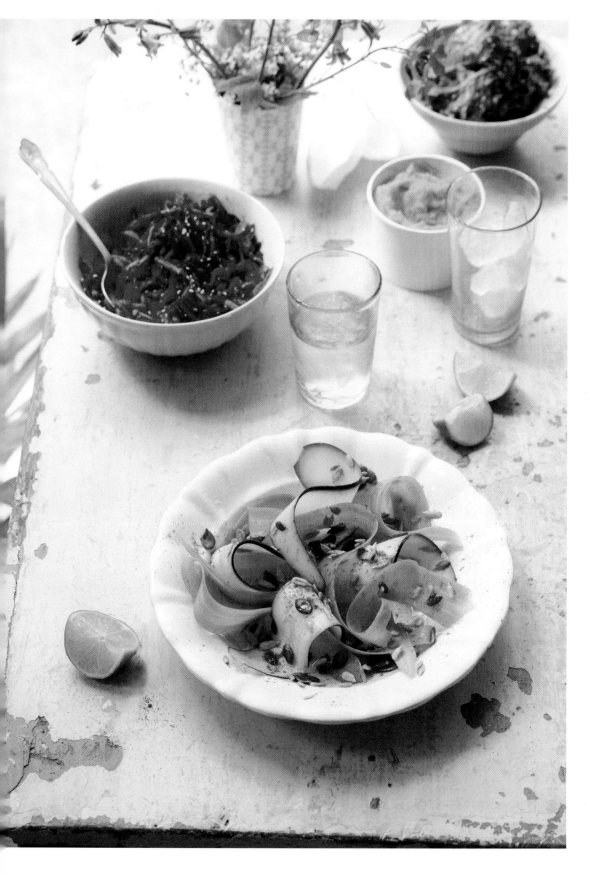

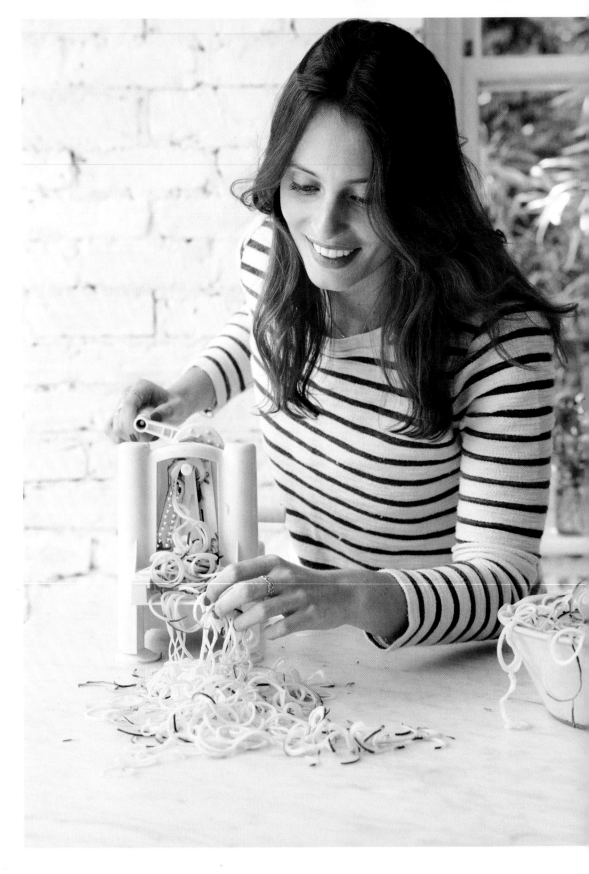

One of my favorite lunch box additions, as it's just bursting with flavor. Zucchini noodles are always a great base for a meal, they're so much more exciting than leaves but are still nice and light. I love mixing this dish with any kind of hummus, my Spiced Squash and Sweet Potato Chunks (pages 66 and 86) and a little arugula.

I have to warn you: these chickpeas are addictive. I normally end up eating the majority of them as soon as they come out of the oven, they're just so good! They make salads delicious. I love a generous handful of them added to my lunch box, as they give a great texture to the meal.

SUN-DRIED TOMATO AND ZUCCHINI NOODLES

Serves 4

2 large zucchini
4 ounces drained oil-packed
    sun-dried tomatoes
2 ounces pine nuts
I cup fresh basil leaves
5 tablespoons olive oil
I garlic clove, roughly chopped
salt and pepper

Use a spiralizer to make the zucchini into noodles. Place them in a large bowl.

Then make the pesto: simply place all the remaining ingredients (not the noodles!) into a food processor, add ½ cup of water and blend until smooth.

Mix the pesto into the noodles. This will keep in the fridge for up to 2 days.

BAKED TOMATO CHICKPEAS

Makes 1 big bowl

two 15-ounce cans chickpeas,
    drained and rinsed
5 ounces drained oil-packed
    sun-dried tomatoes
½ teaspoon chili powder
3 tablespoons olive oil
I tablespoon tomato paste
I tablespoon apple cider vinegar
salt and pepper

Preheat the oven to 350°F (convection 325°F). Put the chickpeas in a mixing bowl.

Add all the remaining ingredients to a food processor and blend until a paste forms; it doesn't have to be totally smooth. Mix thoroughly with the chickpeas, so they're all covered. Spread them out on a large baking sheet; it's important that they have lots of space and aren't sitting on top of each other. Bake for 20–30 minutes, until firm but not crunchy.

Kitchen Know-How

If you can't find sun-dried tomatoes that are simply preserved in olive oil and salt, then soak dry-packed sun-dried tomatoes in boiling water for a couple of minutes, then rinse before using.

A wonderfully simple dish that's all about celebrating natural flavors. The tender veggies mix so well with the homemade sun-dried tomato pesto to create a perfect side dish. I love this in my lunch boxes and as an accompaniment to almost every other meal. It tastes especially amazing with my Chickpea and Squash Salad and Almond Butter Quinoa (pages 96 and 147). It is also a great dish for using up leftovers: simply roast any leftover veggies along with (or instead of) those I have used in this recipe, then mix them with the pesto.

PERFECT PESTO VEGGIES

Serves 3—4

For the veggies

2 eggplants
2 zucchini
2 red bell peppers
olive oil
salt
dried mixed herbs (I use herbes
   de Provence)
handful of fresh basil leaves
   (optional)

For the pesto

12 cherry tomatoes
5 ounces drained oil-packed
   sun-dried tomatoes
1 cup fresh basil leaves
3 tablespoons olive oil
1 tablespoon apple cider vinegar
1 tablespoon tomato paste
1 tablespoon dried herbs
   (I like thyme and oregano)

Preheat the oven to 400°F (convection 350°F).

Cut the eggplants, zucchini and peppers into thin slices and place them on a baking sheet, drizzle with olive oil, salt and dried herbs and roast for 30—40 minutes, flipping everything once or twice during this time.

Meanwhile, make the pesto by simply adding all the ingredients to a food processor, then blending until smooth.

Once the vegetables are cooked and tender, place them in a bowl and mix them up with the pesto, sprinkling with a few more basil leaves, if you like.

Kitchen Know-How

Be generous with your olive oil for the roasted veg, this will make them more tender and stop them from sticking to the pan as they roast.

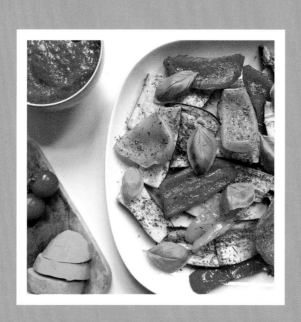

BASIL, THE
FRAGRANCE OF
SUMMER COOKING

This delicious mix of sweet potato and butternut squash is the ultimate addition to any on-the-go meal. It adds a hearty element, while also giving a sweet, comforting touch. The mix goes so well with everything and it's equally delicious hot and cold, so you can also serve it as a side dish to accompany whatever you've chosen as a main. I particularly love dunking the chunks into bowls of Smoky Eggplant Dip or Spicy Turmeric Hummus (pages 65 and 66), it makes the best snack!

SPICED SQUASH AND SWEET POTATO CHUNKS

Serves 4

1 butternut squash
2 large sweet potatoes
2 teaspoons paprika
2 teaspoons dried thyme
2 teaspoons dried oregano
½ teaspoon chili powder
salt
olive oil

Preheat the oven to 425°F (convection 400°F).

Peel the squash (no need to peel the sweet potatoes though), then cut the squash and sweet potatoes into bite-size chunks, about 1 inch square. Place them on a rimmed baking sheet.

Sprinkle the paprika, thyme, oregano, chili powder and salt over the mixture and then drizzle olive oil over everything. Stir it all together until all the chunks are coated in seasoning.

Roast in the oven for 45 minutes to 1 hour, stirring them once or twice during this time to ensure they cook evenly. When you take them out they should be perfectly tender.

Allow to cool, before placing them in an airtight container in the fridge. They will keep in there for up to 4 days.

I first discovered these "fries" when I went out to a dinner and the only thing I could eat was a big bowl of them with hummus. Initially I thought this would be a pretty unexciting meal, but it turns out that it was an amazing combination! For weeks afterward, all I could think about was parsnip fries and hummus, and ever since then I've been making them all the time. I find that they're sweeter than potato wedges and have a nicer texture. They're also stupendous eaten cold.

ROASTED PARSNIP "FRIES"

Serves 2

4 parsnips
olive oil
½ teaspoon ground cumin
½ teaspoon chili flakes
salt and pepper

Preheat the oven to 400°F (convection 350°F).

Slice the parsnips into thin fries.

Drizzle the fries with a generous amount of olive oil, the cumin, chili flakes, salt and pepper.

Place in the oven and bake for up to an hour, turning halfway through, or until they're really nice and tender.

Make It Better

Try mixing parsnip and sweet potato fries; it's an amazing combination! Simply cut the sweet potatoes to the same shape and cook them together.

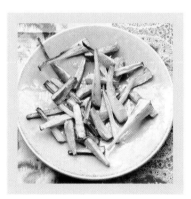

My mom's favorite recipe in the book. We make it a lot together for easy dinners or quick lunches. It's such a simple dish that literally takes three minutes to make, but it really adds so much to a meal as it is so rich in flavor and so vibrant. I love it served with Spicy Turmeric Hummus (page 66), some Spiced Squash and Sweet Potato Chunks (page 86), lots of quinoa and a handful of fresh arugula leaves.

CARROT, BEET AND SESAME SALAD

Serves 3

2 beets
3 carrots
¼ cup sesame seeds
3 tablespoons apple cider vinegar
2 tablespoons maple syrup
salt

Peel the beets and carrots, then grate them using the coarse side of a box grater.

Mix the grated roots in a bowl with the sesame seeds, vinegar, maple syrup and salt. It will keep in the fridge for up to 3 days.

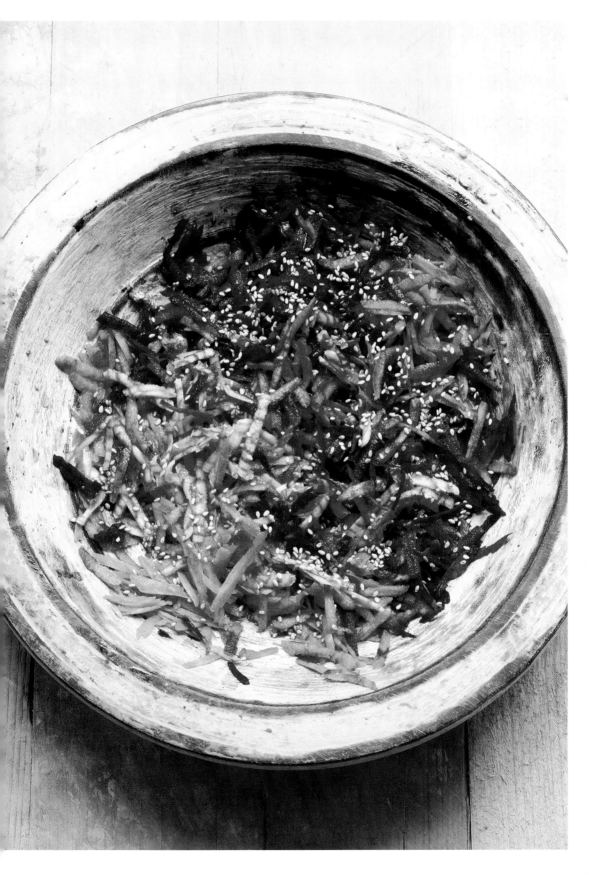

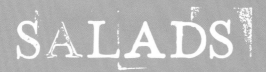

SALADS

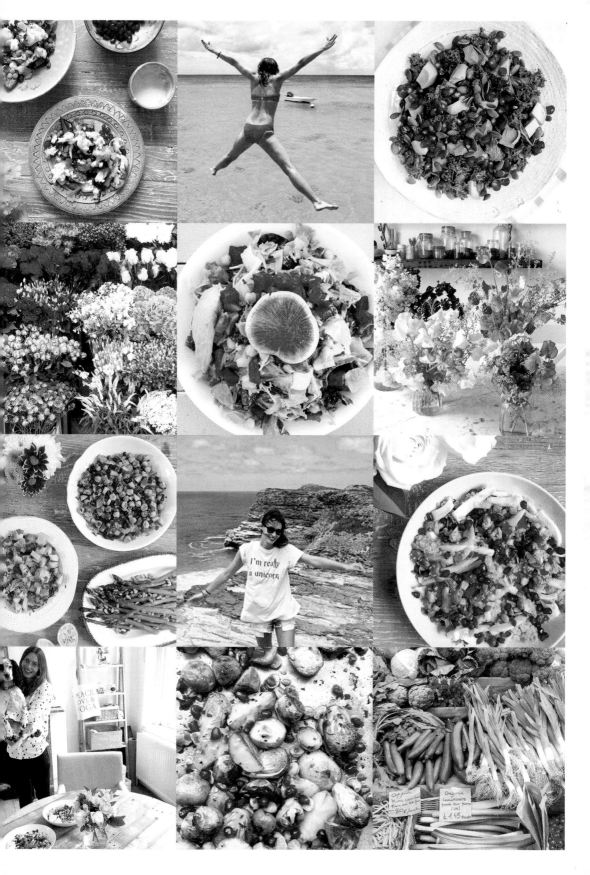

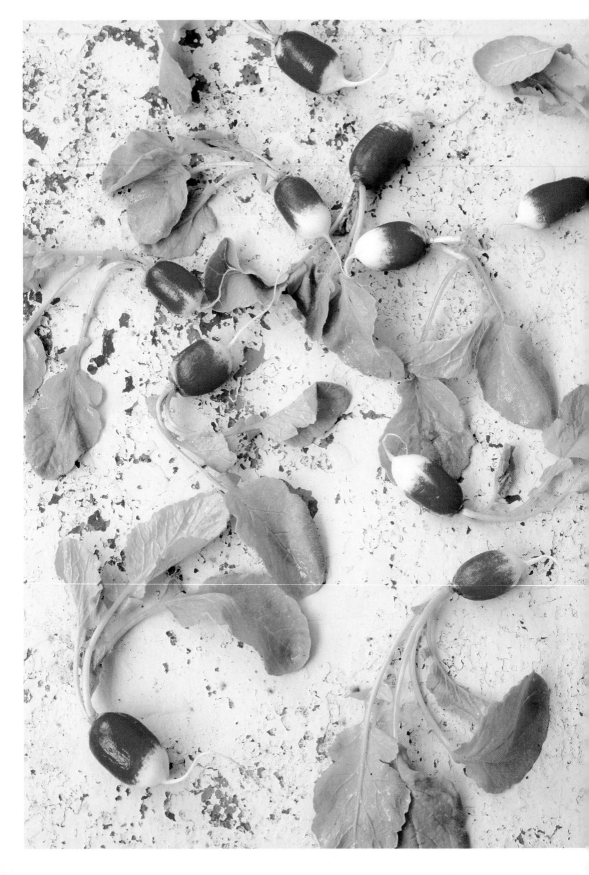

SALADS

I think salads have a bad reputation, which is somewhat unfair. So the aim of this chapter is to reinvent the way we think about them, throw off all the misconceptions and get everyone really excited about enjoying beautiful plates of goodness, because salads really can be the most delicious things in the world.

The word "salad" seems to fill most people with dread, as they imagine plates of iceberg lettuce with soggy cucumber and tomatoes: let's be honest, no one wants to eat that. The number of times I've been to restaurants and they've offered me a plain green salad for dinner is crazy. A plate of green leaves just does not constitute a meal! I think this—coupled with the fact that there is a direct correlation between the words "diet" and "salad"—means very few people get genuinely excited about eating a salad, as they assume it will leave them hungry and uninspired. These feelings are totally justified if you don't make a big, juicy salad that you really adore! It's so important to truly love and enjoy your food, whether it's salad or anything else, as enjoyment is the key to sustainability when it comes to healthy eating.

As I say time and time again, the Deliciously Ella way of eating isn't about a diet, it's about enjoying lots of nourishing, natural food that makes you look and feel your best. So, as we're not trying to restrict ourselves, the kinds of salads you'll see throughout this chapter are abundant, vibrant and hearty. Believe it or not, I actually find that good salads have more texture and flavor than almost any other dish.

I know lots of you may read that sentence and think I am a crazy health freak (which I may be), but I think we're also picturing different salads here. I'm thinking about a huge bowl of chili-roasted chickpeas, tender chunks of butternut squash, juicy sun-dried tomatoes and some peppery arugula all drizzled with a tangy turmeric and honey dressing (page 96); or a plate of cumin-infused wild rice, garlicky cabbage, sweet raisins and a date-based dressing (page 114). Both of these look—and, most importantly, taste—a little different from your average salad.

As you can tell by the descriptions of these two dishes, leaves don't take precedence in my salads. In fact it's the opposite. For me, the leaves are the least important part; the dominant flavor is in the dressing or the other ingredients. So I use salad leaves as a base to add green goodness, or leave them out in favor of a veggie, such as cucumber, or something heartier, such as wild rice or lentils. Lots of my recipes are leaf-free yet oh-so-delicious, from Middle Eastern–Inspired Salad (page 100) to Simple Cucumber and Tomato Salad (page 104) and Roasted Maple Sprouts (page 116). I think you'll find, once you decrease the leaf ratio, you will have something more delicious, no matter what the other ingredients are!

You don't have to omit leaves entirely. I include greens in lots of meals; they're full of the vitamins and minerals that keep me feeling great. I'm just saying you don't need to put all the emphasis on lettuce or other leaves; see them simply as one ingredient in a mélange of beautiful things, rather than the centerpiece. The salads in this chapter that do contain leaves tend to be a little lighter, so they're great for the days when you're not especially hungry, or want to serve salad as a side dish. For these days, we have recipes such as Wilted Spinach and Black Bean Salad; or Winter Kale Salad with a wonderfully creamy tahini dressing, sweet apple and grated beet; or Mango and Avocado Salsa (pages 98, 110, and 112).

The other core component of a salad is the dressing, which I think is the most important part. Dressings bring ingredients together, making each bite taste amazing. Simple olive oil dressings are great, but in just a minute we can create something far more exciting to spice up your plate: think creamy garlic and tahini; sesame oil and honey; spicy chili and tamari; or sweet almond and maple. I mean, how good do they all sound? Drizzle one of those amazing concoctions over your salad and it will instantly spring to life. (Keep the dressing in a small pot when you are packing up your salad for lunch and pour it over at the last minute for maximum deliciousness.) Each recipe comes with a different dressing, but all share ingredients that you can keep in stock so you always have them handy.

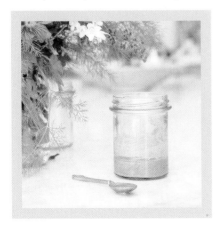

KEY DRESSING INGREDIENTS

Olive oil—the base of all my dressings. There's a huge variety in the oils you can buy, both in taste and price. I buy organic extra virgin and like to spend a little more to buy a nicer bottle, as it adds so much flavor to a dressing. To save money, try keeping two bottles: a cheaper oil to use in cooking, as you don't really taste it, and a more expensive one with a richer flavor for dressings and to drizzle over food.

Apple cider vinegar—a great alternative to balsamic vinegar as it is very alkalizing and amazing for digestive issues. I use it in a lot of salad dressings as it has a delicious tangy flavor that really livens them up. I normally use either vinegar or lemon/lime juice as the acid component, because the two together can be a little too tangy.

Honey/maple syrup—I sweeten dressings with these. A little goes a long way, as the sweetness shouldn't be overpowering, just a teaspoon or so. If you're trying to avoid sweeteners, leave them out and the dressing will still be delicious. If you're vegan, swap the honey for maple syrup. I buy raw honey as it has more health benefits and a stronger, more delicious flavor, but any will work. With maple syrup, check you're buying a pure syrup, as supermarkets can sell syrups that are only ten percent maple and as much as ninety percent additives and flavorings!

Garlic—I never used to eat garlic as it didn't agree with my stomach, but over the last few years I've slowly reintroduced it and now my body loves it, which is such a blessing as it's so delicious! Garlic adds so much great flavor to a dressing. I normally add it raw as I love how strong and almost hot the flavor is, plus it has amazing heath benefits; but you can add roasted garlic instead, which has a much mellower flavor.

Herbs and spices—essential in most dressings and for just about everything else. In dressings, I especially love chili flakes . . .

Lemon or lime juice—the easiest way to freshen up a salad. The citrusy flavors complement all the other ingredients here (except the vinegar), so you can add them to any combination. Lime is sweeter than lemon and normally has a weaker flavor, so I use it when I want a citrus flavor to blend into the dressing, and I choose lemon when I want the taste to stand out.

Sesame oil—my new favorite way to add flavor to just about everything. It's wonderful in dressings. It has a subtle flavor that's hard to pinpoint, but really adds something magical!

Tamari—one of the best ingredients for salad dressings as it makes them so rich, which means each bite bursts with flavor. Tamari has quite a salty taste, so you won't need to add much salt to a dressing if it includes tamari. If you don't have any tamari at home you can use soy sauce instead as they're pretty much the same; tamari is just usually gluten-free (though check the bottle) and normally has no additives or sugar.

Tahini and almond butter—both work wonders in a dressing, giving a creamy texture. Almond butter is a lot nuttier than tahini and tahini is slightly more bitter, but neither flavor is overpowering and they're primarily used for their textures, so are pretty interchangeable in dressings. If you have a nut allergy, use tahini instead.

SHOPPING LIST

ALMOND BUTTER

APPLE CIDER VINEGAR

ARUGULA

AVOCADOS

BASIL

BEETS

BLACK BEANS

BUCKWHEAT NOODLES

BUTTERNUT SQUASH

CILANTRO

CUCUMBER

GARLIC

GREEN BEANS

HONEY

LEMONS

LIMES

MANGOES

MAPLE SYRUP

MINT

OLIVE OIL

PEPPERS

POMEGRANATES

RAISINS

RED CABBAGE

SESAME OIL

SWEET POTATOES

TAHINI

TAMARI

WILD RICE

This may sound simple but—trust me—it's so much more than it seems. I first made this for a collaboration with a café in London and it was such a hit that I knew I had to share it with you all, too! It is a great simple dinner for one, or you can make a huge bowl of it to serve with friends alongside lots of my Black Bean Burgers (page 182).

CHICKPEA AND SQUASH SALAD

Serves 1

For the salad

4-ounce chunk of butternut
   squash
1 teaspoon paprika
1 teaspoon dried mixed herbs
   (I use herbes de Provence)
salt
olive oil
½ cup canned chickpeas,
   drained and rinsed
½ teaspoon chili powder
big handful of arugula (about
   2 ounces)
1½ ounces drained oil-packed
   sun-dried tomatoes, chopped

For the dressing

1 tablespoon olive oil
½ tablespoon apple cider vinegar
½ teaspoon ground turmeric
1 teaspoon honey
salt and pepper

Preheat the oven to 425°F (convection 400°F).

Peel the squash, then cut it into small bite-size pieces. Place on a baking sheet with the paprika, mixed herbs, a little salt and olive oil. Bake for about 30 minutes, until tender.

Place the chickpeas on a separate baking sheet with the chili powder, toss well to coat and bake for 20 minutes, until they're firm but not too crunchy.

Mix all the dressing ingredients together, seasoning with a bit of salt and lots of pepper.

Once the chickpeas and squash have cooked and cooled, mix them with the arugula and sun-dried tomatoes, then pour on the dressing and toss everything together.

Tweak It

If you don't have any squash, then try using sweet potato instead, it tastes awesome in this.

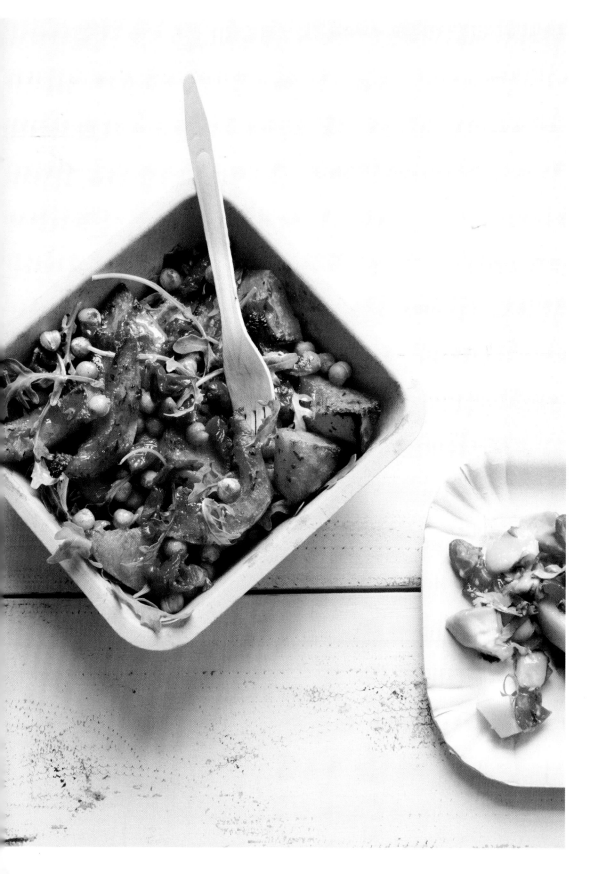

Such a winner if you're looking for a simple, nourishing dish to warm you up! The roasted squash and zucchini taste amazing with the sautéed beans and spinach, then the creamy tahini and miso dressing just bring it all together. If I'm not especially hungry I love this just as it is, but if you want to make it a little heartier, serve it over quinoa or brown rice. That's delicious.

WILTED SPINACH AND BLACK BEAN SALAD

Serves 1

For the salad

⅓ butternut squash
olive oil
salt and pepper
½ zucchini
3 ounces spinach
¾ cup canned black beans,
    drained and rinsed

For the dressing

1 tablespoon tahini
2 tablespoons olive oil
⅓ teaspoon chili powder
½ teaspoon ground cumin
1 teaspoon miso paste
juice of ½ lemon

Preheat the oven to 400°F (convection 350°F).

Peel the squash, then cut it into bite-size pieces. Place these on a baking sheet with a little olive oil, salt and pepper. Bake for 30 minutes, until tender.

Cut the zucchini into thin half moons. After the squash has cooked for 20 minutes, add the zucchini to the baking sheet to roast alongside for the last 10 minutes.

While the zucchini and squash finish cooking, place the spinach and beans in a frying pan with a little olive oil and gently sauté them. Add the zucchini and squash once they come out of the oven. Let everything cook together while you mix all the ingredients for the dressing.

Pour the dressing over the salad, mix it well, then serve.

Shop Sense

To save on money and food wastage, cut up the whole squash and roast it along with the other veggies you need here, then use the leftover squash in your meals over the next few days.

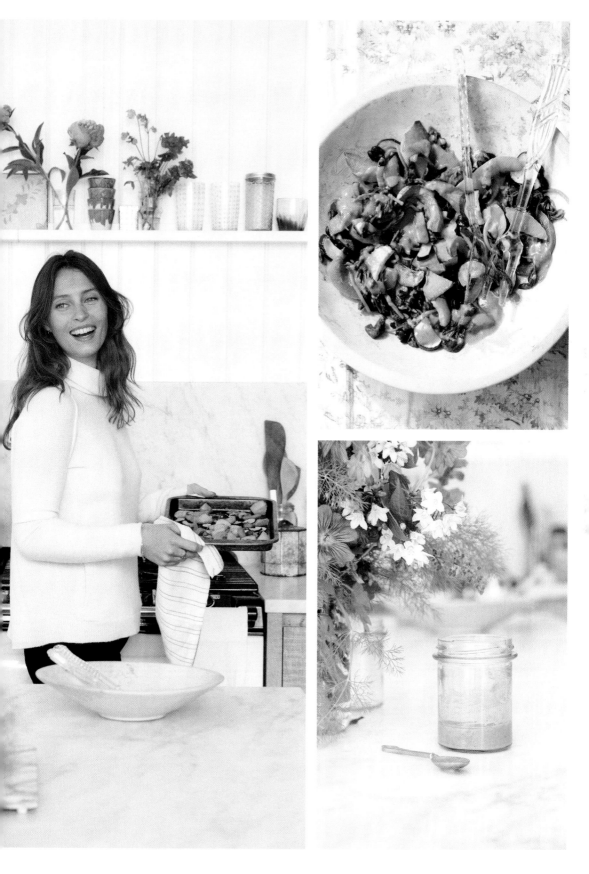

This Ottolenghi-inspired dish is full of delicious Middle Eastern flavors. The roasted cauliflower, eggplant and lentils mix so well with lots of sweet pomegranates, cilantro and a creamy dressing of tahini and vinegar. The result is pretty magical!

MIDDLE EASTERN–INSPIRED SALAD

Serves 6

For the salad

1 cauliflower
2 eggplants
2 teaspoons tamari
olive oil
salt and pepper
generous ½ cup Puy lentils
½ cup cilantro leaves,
    finely chopped
generous 1 cup pomegranate
    seeds

For the dressing

3 tablespoons olive oil
1 tablespoon apple cider vinegar
2 tablespoons tahini
2 garlic cloves, crushed

Preheat the oven to 350°F (convection 325°F).

Chop the cauliflower and eggplants into bite-size pieces and place them on a large baking sheet with half the tamari, some olive oil, salt and pepper. Bake for 30 minutes.

Next, place the lentils into a saucepan with the remaining tamari and 2 cups of boiling water. Place the lid on the pan and bring the lentils to a boil again, then reduce the heat to a simmer and cook for about 20 minutes, until all the water has been absorbed.

Meanwhile, mix together all the ingredients for the dressing and let them sit for a while so the flavors can infuse.

Allow the cauliflower, eggplant and lentils to cool down for a few minutes, then combine them all in a salad bowl with the dressing, mixing gently.

Sprinkle with the cilantro and pomegranate seeds and mix so everything is lightly coated in the dressing, then serve.

Kitchen Know-How

Make sure to use a large baking sheet to roast the cauliflower and eggplants, or they'll all sit on top of each other and become a little soggy.

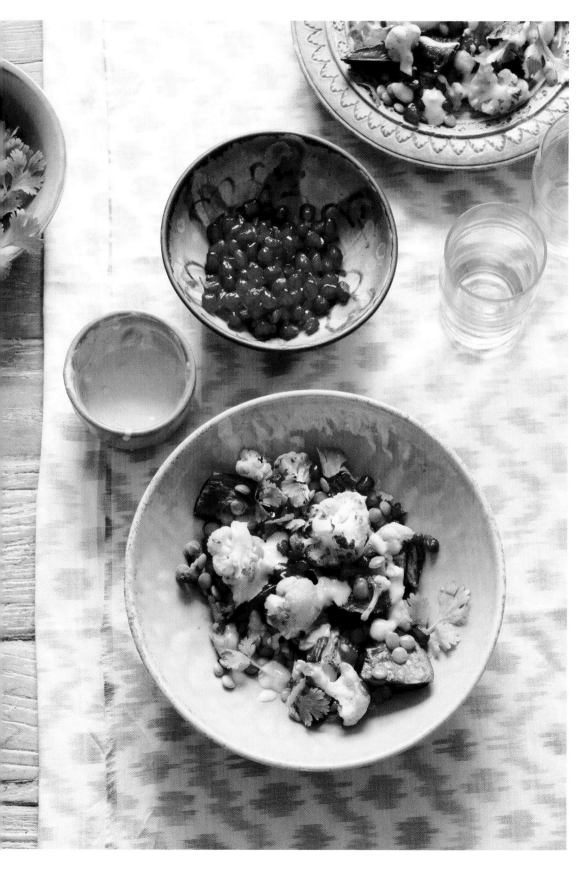

Perhaps not the most beautiful dish in the book, but I promise it's still so delicious! Using hummus as the dressing means it's creamy, while the vinegar adds a subtle tanginess to each bite. I love this served with Mango and Avocado Salsa (page 112) and a little quinoa; it's a dreamy combination!

SAUTÉED POTATO, KALE AND HUMMUS

Serves 4

6 baby potatoes (½ pound)
salt and pepper
olive oil
1 teaspoon chili flakes
5 big handfuls of kale (5 ounces)
7 ounces cherry tomatoes
7 ounces jarred oil-packed
   artichoke hearts (a drained
   9.9-ounce jar)
2 teaspoons apple cider vinegar
5 tablespoons hummus, ideally
   Spicy Turmeric Hummus
   (page 66)

Place the potatoes in a pan of cold salted water and bring to a boil, then reduce the heat and let them simmer for 20 minutes, until they're soft enough to pierce with a fork. Drain the potatoes, rinse them with cold water and, once they're cool enough to handle, cut them into thin slices.

Heat a little olive oil in a large frying pan and fry the potato slices with the chili flakes and some salt and pepper for 2 minutes, to give them a little color.

Rip the kale into pieces, removing the coarse stems, then place the leaves in the frying pan with the potatoes. Cook until the kale wilts, stirring every now and again.

Chop the tomatoes in half and add these to the frying pan. Cook for another 5 minutes.

Finally, chop the artichokes into bite-size pieces and add these to the pan with the vinegar and hummus. Stir everything together, then serve.

Kitchen Know-How

This dish is nicest served hot and fresh. It's one of the few meals where leftovers aren't as good as the original, so just make the amount you need for a single meal.

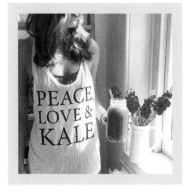

The perfect side salad for any meal. It's simple and goes with anything, but the flavors and textures are so much more exciting than those of a classic green salad. The sweet potato makes it more filling, while the oven-roasted tomatoes add a sweet, juicy element to each bite of peppery arugula. I love this served with my Zucchini and Carrot Strip Salad (page 80), the two go so well together!

SWEET POTATO AND ARUGULA

Serves 2

For the salad

1 large sweet potato
1 tablespoon mixed dried herbs
salt
olive oil
12 cherry tomatoes
3.5 ounces arugula leaves

For the dressing

2 tablespoons olive oil
1 tablespoon apple cider vinegar
salt and pepper

Preheat the oven to 425°F (convection 400°F).

Slice the sweet potato into wedges. Place the wedges on a baking sheet with the dried herbs, a sprinkling of salt and a drizzling of olive oil, tossing to coat. Put in the oven and cook for about 45 minutes, until they're nice and tender.

Meanwhile, cut the cherry tomatoes in half. About 10 minutes before the sweet potatoes finish cooking, add the tomatoes to the baking sheet with an extra drizzling of olive oil and let these cook until they're very juicy and soft.

Once the tomatoes and sweet potatoes have finished cooking, remove them from the oven and leave to cool.

Toss the arugula in a salad bowl with all the ingredients for the dressing. Then add the sweet potato wedges and tomatoes to the salad and gently toss once more to serve.

I know the ingredients list for this recipe sounds too incredibly simple, but the end result is unbelievably fantastic! It's the simplicity that makes this salad great, as the flavor and texture of each individual ingredient really stand out. It's a very light, fresh-tasting combination, too, so it's the perfect addition to any meal, as it really goes with absolutely everything. It also only takes five minutes to make, which is great if you need a speedy side dish to impress your dinner guests.

SIMPLE CUCUMBER AND TOMATO SALAD

Serves 4 (as a side dish)

5 ounces cherry tomatoes
1 large cucumber
6 tablespoons pine nuts
juice of 1 lime
1 tablespoon olive oil
salt and pepper

Cut the cherry tomatoes into quarters.

Slice the cucumber lengthwise into 8 pieces, then slice the seedy center out of all of them (discard this). Chop the cucumber into thin pieces.

Place the pine nuts in a dry frying pan and let them cook, stirring, for 2–3 minutes, until they turn a golden brown.

Mix the pine nuts, tomatoes and cucumber together in a bowl, then add the lime juice, olive oil, salt and lots of pepper.

Kitchen Know-How

Be careful toasting the pine nuts: they seem to go from raw to burnt in 30 seconds . . . keep an eye on them!

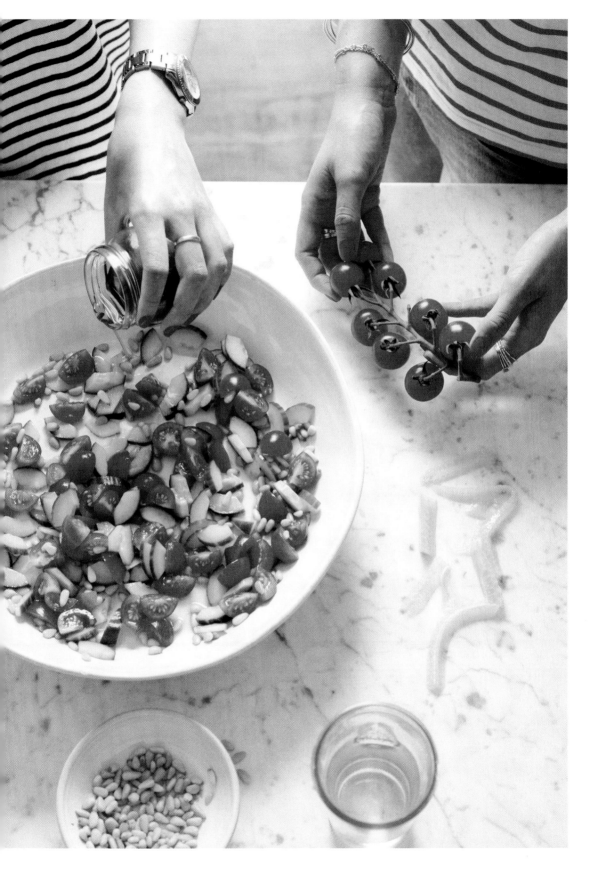

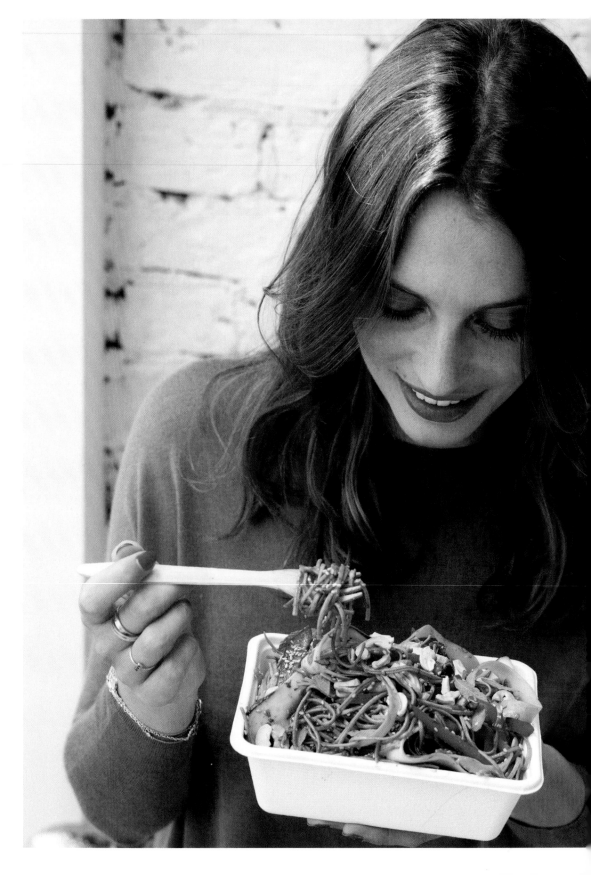

Such a delicious dish, I think it may end up being a favorite recipe for lots of you . . . it's certainly very popular in my house! It's inspired by a recipe that a friend sent to me; I fell in love with it and adapted it over time to create this version. The sauce is definitely my favorite part, as it's so incredibly rich with the most amazing array of flavors.

PAD THAI

Serves 2

For the noodles

2 large zucchini
2 large carrots
3.5 ounces buckwheat noodles
1 red bell pepper, cut into
   very thin strips
handful of sesame seeds
1 ounce cashew nuts
¼ cup fresh mint leaves,
   finely chopped

For the sauce

½ cup olive oil
½ cup bunch of cilantro
3 tablespoons almond butter
2 tablespoons tahini
1 tablespoon maple syrup
1 tablespoon tamari
juice of 1 lemon
3 garlic cloves, crushed
1 teaspoon cayenne pepper

Peel the zucchini, then use a vegetable peeler to peel the flesh into strips around the core. I normally discard the seedy centers, as they're hard to peel. Do the same with the carrots.

Cook the noodles according to the package instructions.

Meanwhile, make the sauce. Simply place everything into a blender or food processer with ½ cup plus 1 tablespoon of water and blend until smooth.

Once the noodles have cooked, drain them and let them cool for a few minutes.

Place the noodles, carrots, zucchini, bell pepper, sesame seeds and cashews in a large bowl and pour over the dressing. Mix everything together, then sprinkle the mint on top.

Tweak It

For a lighter salad, skip the buckwheat noodles and use an extra zucchini and carrot instead.

This awesome salad takes just ten minutes to make and it's totally fuss-free! It's so easy to throw together and there are no complicated steps, so even the newest cook will be able to ace it. It's a wonderful dish to serve as a side as it doesn't have any strong, overpowering flavors: instead the mix of beans, tomatoes, pine nuts, basil, lime and sesame seeds subtly blends into any main dish, adding great textures and extra goodness. It's especially good with the Creamy Sweet Potato or Mushroom Risotto (pages 176 and 184) and, as shown here, with other salads as part of a lunch box.

GREEN BEANS AND SALSA

Serves 6 (as a side dish)

1 pound green beans
4 large tomatoes
6 tablespoons pine nuts
handful of fresh basil leaves
⅓ cup sesame seeds
juice of 2 limes
¼ cup olive oil
salt and pepper

Cut the ends from the beans, then chop them into thirds. Place these in a steamer and steam for 10 minutes until they're ever so slightly crunchy, but soft enough to eat.

Meanwhile, chop the tomatoes, discarding the seedy centers.

Toast the pine nuts in a dry frying pan for a minute or so, until they smell toasty and turn a shade darker.

Finely chop the basil leaves.

Place the tomatoes in a bowl with the toasted pine nuts, basil, sesame seeds, lime juice, olive oil, salt and pepper. Add the beans once they're cooked, then stir everything together.

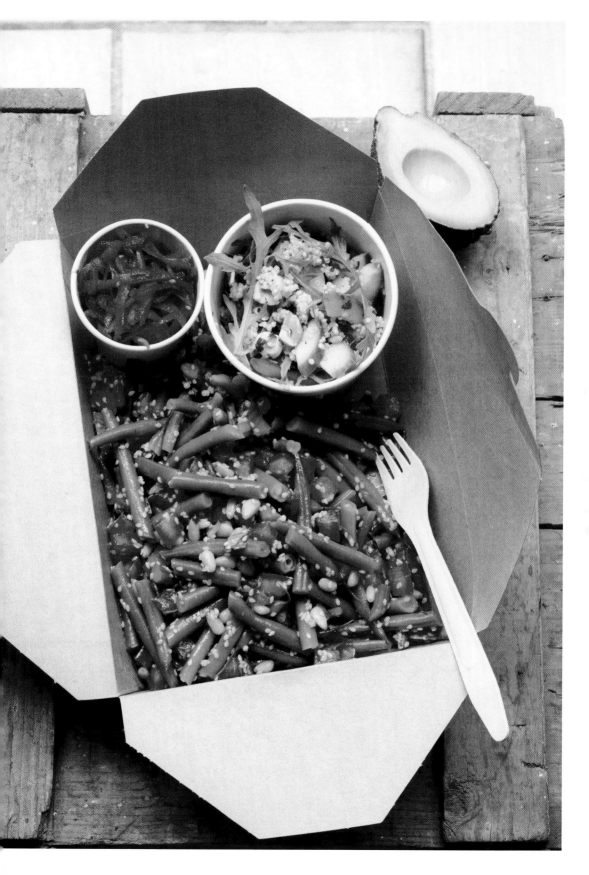

My favorite cold–weather salad! We made it in my cooking classes last winter and it was such a hit. The dark green kale with bright purple beet is beautiful, a feast for the eyes as well as the stomach. I love it with Creamy Sweet Potato Risotto, or My Favorite Sweet Potato Cakes (pages 176 and 189).

WINTER KALE SALAD

Serves 4

9 ounces kale
juice of 2 limes
¼ cup tahini
3 tablespoons tamari
2 tablespoons olive oil
2 beets
2 apples
¾ cup pine nuts
salt and pepper

Tear the kale leaves from their stems and put into a salad bowl. Add the lime juice, tahini, tamari and olive oil.

Use your hands to firmly massage the kale with the dressing, really working it into each leaf. After a couple of minutes you should feel the kale start to wilt and soften.

Peel the beets and apples, then grate them using the coarse side of a box grater.

Place the pine nuts in a small frying pan and dry-fry for a couple of minutes until lightly toasted.

Add the pine nuts, grated apple and beet to the kale and mix everything together, seasoning well with salt and pepper.

Kitchen Know–How

If you're leaving this in the fridge for awhile, add a little extra lime or lemon juice to stop the apple from turning brown.

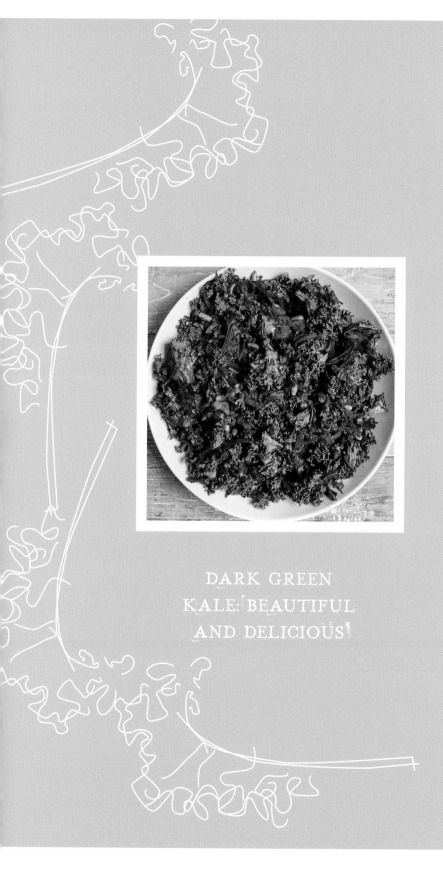

DARK GREEN
KALE: BEAUTIFUL
AND DELICIOUS

An amazing salad if you want to impress anyone! It's full of such incredible flavors that liven up any dish. I love using it as a bed to serve a main course upon, as it adds a wonderful sweetness while also making the meal look so delicious because the colors are so vibrant. The lime juice and tomatoes add a wonderful freshness, while the avocado and olive oil make the salad a little creamy.

MANGO AND AVOCADO SALSA

Serves 4

2 mangoes
2 avocados
7 ounces cherry tomatoes
small handful of cilantro leaves,
    finely chopped
juice of 1 lime
3 tablespoons olive oil
salt

Peel the mangoes, then chop them into small pieces.

Cut the avocados in half, remove the pits and cut the flesh into pieces the same size as the mango.

Cut the cherry tomatoes into eighths.

Mix the mangoes, avocados, tomatoes and cilantro in a bowl, then add the lime juice, olive oil and salt. Toss to serve.

Kitchen Know-How

If you want to keep this in the fridge for a few days, don't add the avocado until just before eating. This will help it stay fresher for longer.

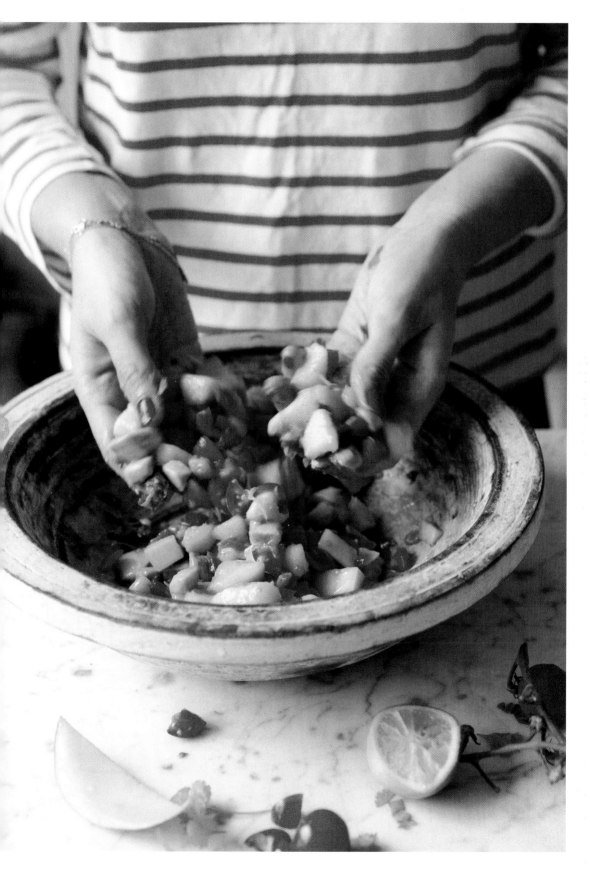

The ideal winter salad; it's warming and comforting and goes with everything. It's inspired by my mom, who cooks the best cabbage at home, so I thought I would expand on her recipe and add the rice, raisins and dressing to make something even more delicious! The cumin and sesame seeds give it a wonderful flavor and the raisins lend it a sweet, juicy bite. I love serving this with some Roasted Parsnip "Fries" and my Middle Eastern—Inspired Salad (pages 87 and 100): a delicious meal!

SWEET WILD RICE, CABBAGE AND SESAME

Serves 4

2 red apples
1 red cabbage, cored and chopped
2 tablespoons apple cider vinegar
⅔ cup raisins
salt
scant 1 cup wild rice
2 tablespoons date syrup
1 tablespoon cumin seeds
juice of ½ lemon
1 tablespoon tahini
½ cup sesame seeds

Peel and core the apples and cut them into bite-size pieces. Place in a saucepan with the cabbage and ⅔ cup of boiling water. Add the vinegar, raisins and a little salt. Bring to a boil, then reduce the heat to a simmer and cook for 1 hour.

Meanwhile, cook the wild rice according to the package instructions.

When the cabbage has cooked for an hour, add the wild rice, date syrup, cumin, lemon juice and a little more salt. Let everything simmer together for a final 5 minutes.

When ready to serve, take it off the heat and mix in the tahini and sesame seeds.

Make It Better

If you're eating this salad on its own and want to boost the protein intake, try adding some cannellini beans.

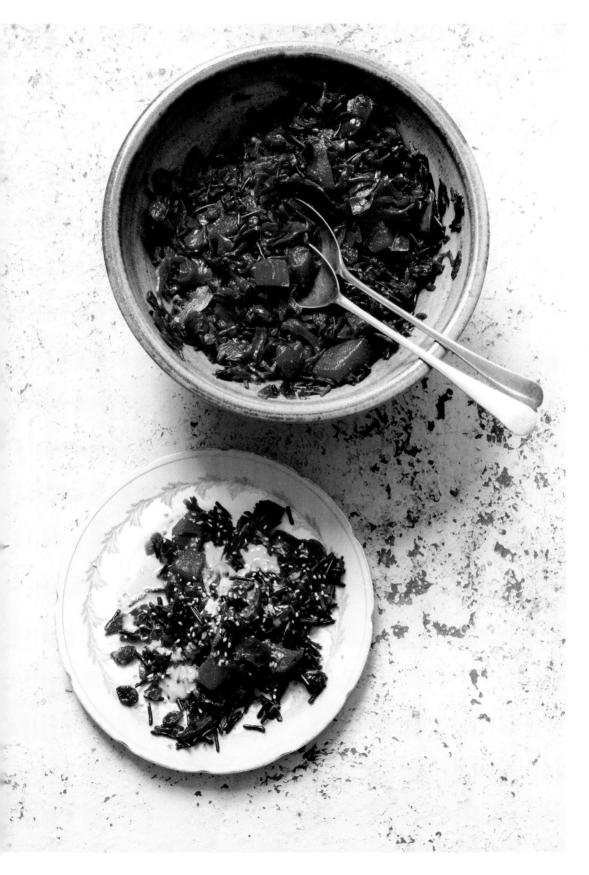

I know Brussels sprouts aren't the most popular vegetable out there, but—trust me—this dish will revolutionize the way you look at them! Baking sprouts turns them so crispy, which instantly changes the way they taste. When combined with chili-infused potatoes, crunchy hazelnuts, juicy pomegranates and a sweet maple dressing, you'll instantly forget any preconceptions you have and fall totally in love with sprouts.

ROASTED MAPLE SPROUTS

Serves 4

7 ounces Brussels sprouts
8 new potatoes
1 teaspoon chili flakes
olive oil
salt and pepper
2 ounces blanched hazelnuts
½ cup pomegranate seeds
2 tablespoons maple syrup

Preheat the oven to 400°F (convection 350°F).

Halve the sprouts lengthwise and cut the potatoes into pieces roughly the same size as the sprouts.

Place the sprouts and potatoes on a baking dish with the chili flakes and a drizzling of olive oil, salt and pepper. Bake for about 30 minutes, until they start to turn a golden brown.

Add the hazelnuts, toss everything about, then roast the dish for another 10 minutes, until the nuts are golden brown, too.

Take the baking dish out the oven and stir the pomegranate seeds into the mixture. Drizzle the maple syrup and 2 tablespoons of olive oil over everything and mix well.

Make It Better

Serve this at Christmas to convince everyone else how amazing sprouts are! A big bowl of this salad will prove a serious upgrade from traditional boiled sprouts.

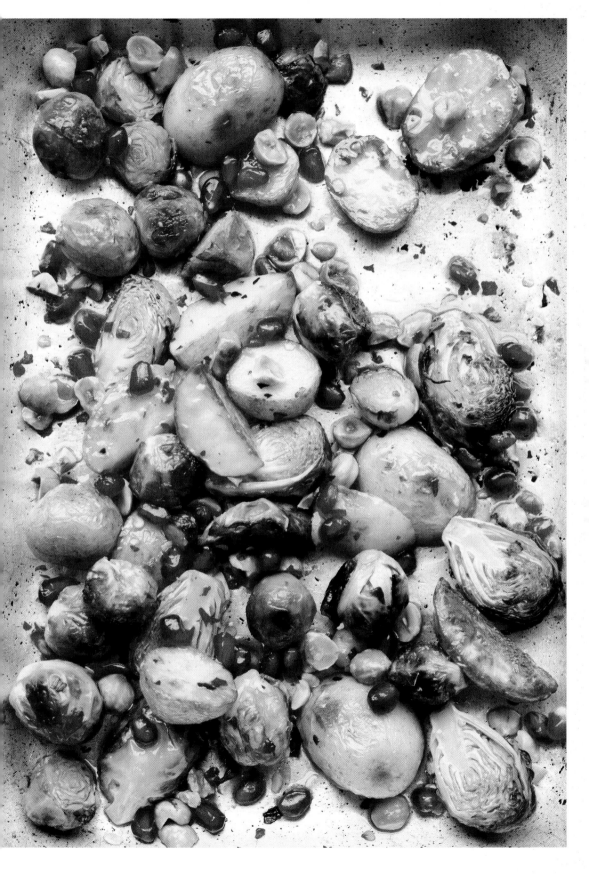

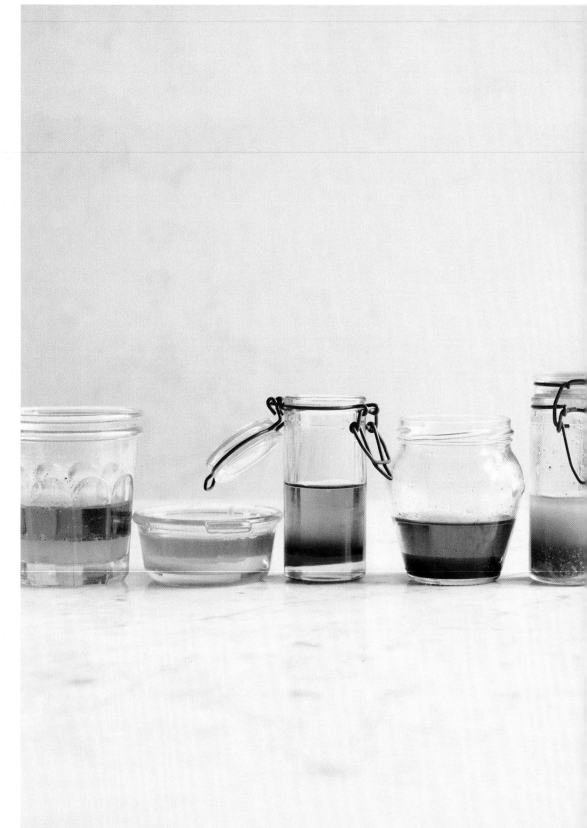

Dressings are a really important part of eating well, as they instantly spice up any meal. I add them to all my salads, roasted veggies, grains, beans and anything else I cook. The simple lime and olive oil mix here is the best dressing for an easy side salad; the flavors are subtle and easily blend with whatever you're eating. The garlic and tahini version is the creamiest, so I love using it with grains and sautéed beans to create a rich dish. The sweet sesame is probably my favorite, the flavors are just so incredible, it's similar to the almond and maple dressing but the almond version is much creamier whereas the sesame dressing is a little lighter. The chili and tamari is the richest, with a delicious mix of saltiness and spice that really strengthens the flavors of whatever you pair it with.

EASY SALAD DRESSINGS, FIVE WAYS

All dress a side salad for 2

SIMPLE LIME AND OLIVE OIL
juice of 1 lime
3 tablespoons olive oil
1 teaspoon apple cider vinegar
salt and pepper

GARLIC AND TAHINI
2 garlic cloves, crushed or finely grated
3 tablespoons olive oil
1 heaping tablespoon tahini
juice of ½ lime
salt

SWEET SESAME
2 teaspoons sesame oil
2 tablespoons olive oil
1 teaspoon maple syrup

ALMOND AND MAPLE
1 heaping teaspoon almond butter
1 teaspoon maple syrup
2 tablespoons olive oil

CHILI AND TAMARI
1 teaspoon tamari
sprinkling of chili powder
3 tablespoons olive oil
juice of ½ lime
salt

EASY WEEKDAY DINNERS

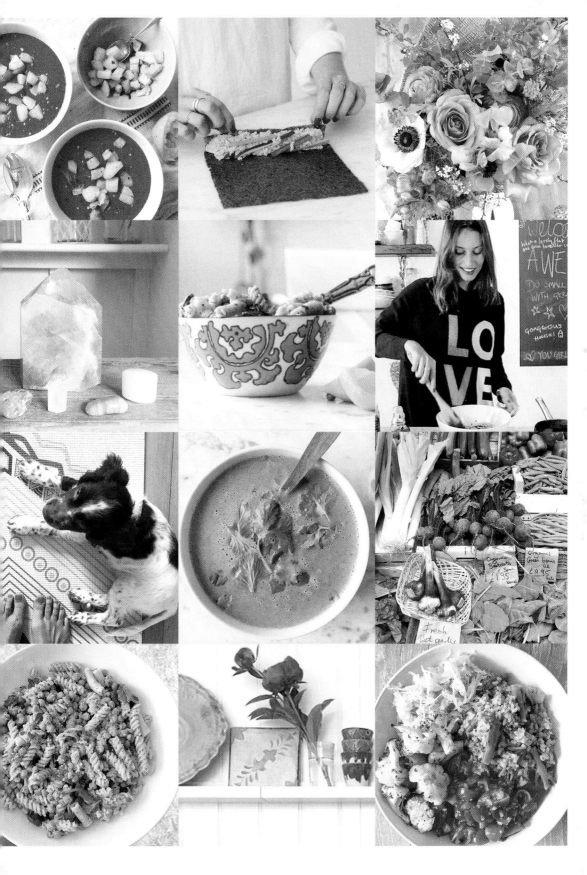

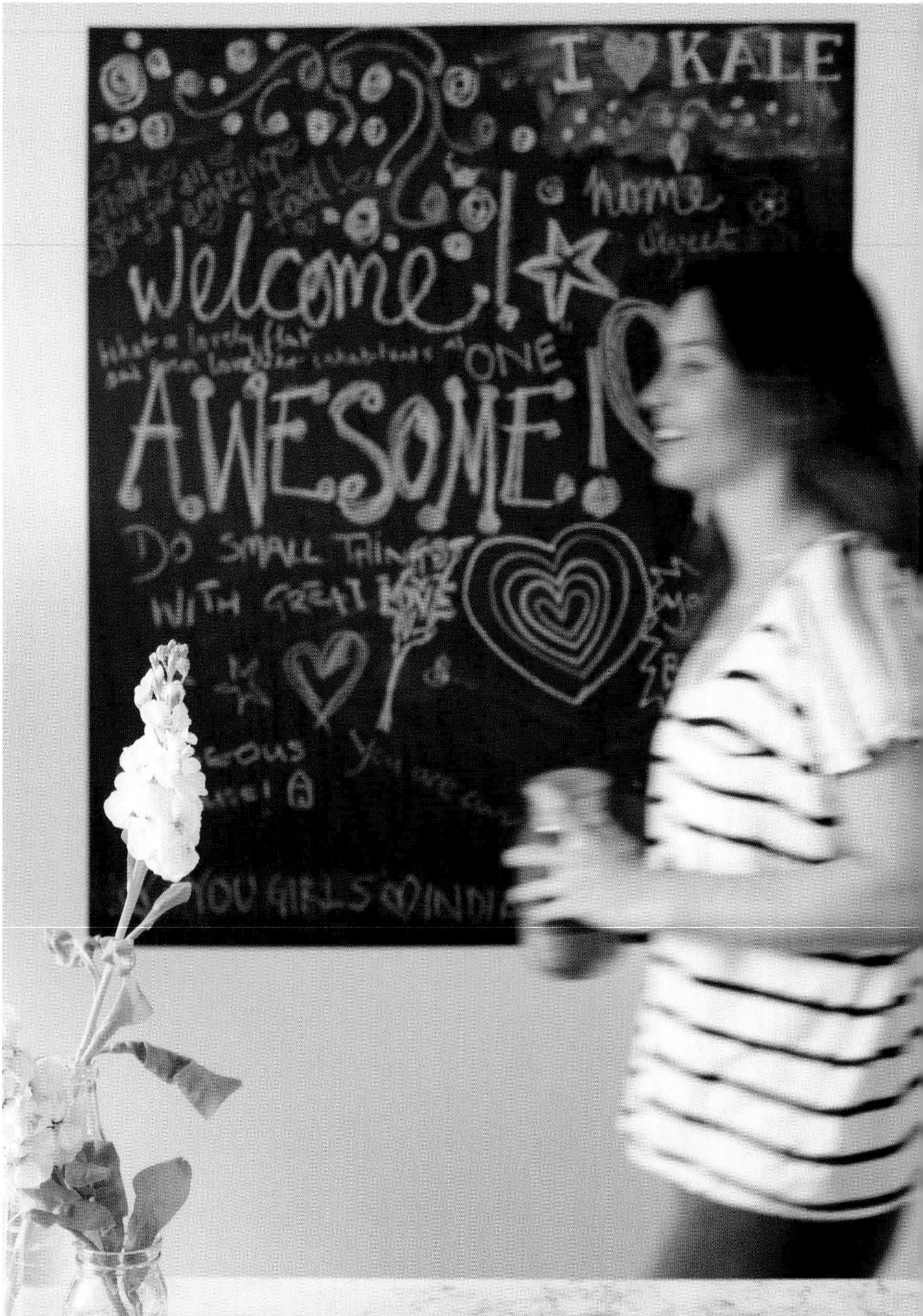
KALE
welcome!
ONE
AWESOME!
home

EASY WEEKDAY DINNERS

The recipes over the next few pages are designed to nurture, soothe and energize you after a long day, so you feel like a whole new person by the time you finish your plate. I use them when I'm at home on my own or if I'm making a chilled kitchen supper to catch up with a couple of close friends. Each dish is delightfully easy to throw together but, rest assured, although they may be simple to make, they taste absolutely divine and—what's more— you can keep some for lunch the next day. Trust me: both you and your guests will be very impressed. I mean, who wouldn't love a baked sweet potato stuffed with garlic mushrooms, sautéed black beans, soft avocado chunks and a sweet tahini dressing (page 145); or perhaps a comforting bowl of Bright Pink Soup with chili-infused potato croutons (page 128)? You'll look and feel like a domestic goddess by the end of the meal, I promise!

To make each dish even simpler, I've avoided using hard-to-find ingredients or costly equipment, so you should be able to cook almost everything in this chapter in any kitchen anywhere in the world. The vast majority of ingredients should be available in your local supermarket, so you shouldn't need to go to a special shop. You also won't need a food processor for most of the recipes. The soups will of course need a blender, but a simple handheld version is perfect. There are only two recipes that may need something a little stronger for blending and, in both of those, substitutions can be made if you don't have a powerful blender or food processor.

The pesto in the Warming Pesto Lima Beans (page 157) can be replaced with store-bought pesto, for example, while the avocado cream in the Quinoa Nori Rolls (page 158) can be replaced with mashed avocado; both will still taste delicious after these little swaps, so please don't rule them out if your kitchen kit is not up to scratch! Apart from these two, everything else just requires pots, pans, spoons, knives, bowls and a good appetite.

The other great thing about these recipes is that they're wonderfully inexpensive, as they focus on really simple ingredients: veggies, beans, pulses, grains and spices. There aren't even many nuts or seeds involved, so the cost of each bowlful should be very low. That's the thing about a plant-based diet, people assume it's expensive, because prepackaged products in health food stores are pricey but, in reality, what I eat on a daily basis costs very little.

A bowl of roasted eggplant slices with brown rice, sautéed spinach, garlicky beans and a tahini dressing (page 140) is not an expensive dish to make, nor is a bowl of comforting lentils and potatoes in a homemade tomato sauce (page 151); both will fill you with goodness and taste wonderful, but they absolutely won't break the bank. You will find that if you eat something like that for dinner, some overnight oats for breakfast and a quinoa bowl with a tahini dressing and kale for lunch, you will spend relatively little in the short term but will enrich your body with so much goodness and nourishment, which is, I think, a great long-term investment. It's so important to invest in your health; it may mean spending a bit more time, energy and money on your meals to start with, but in the long run it's completely worth it.

Another idea if you're looking to keep costs down is to focus on buying seasonal, local produce. As it doesn't travel far, the price will be lower, so choosing apples rather than mangoes, pears rather than pineapples and kale rather than bok choy will make a huge difference to your budget all year round. In winter, focus on recipes that use winter roots (carrots, beets, sweet potatoes and so on); in summer, enjoy the recipes filled with peppers, asparagus and tomatoes. You don't have to only cook seasonally, you just may find that it's kinder on your wallet.

What are we going to cook over the next few pages? We're going to start with awesome soups. Then we'll look at easy veggie recipes, such as roasted cauliflower with lime-infused peas and asparagus, and my sisters' favorite mashed potato bowl with broccoli, zucchini and corn (pages 137 and 152). Finally, we'll move to grain- and bean-centered dishes, such as Green Goodness Bowl with miso- and lemon-infused veggies and my favorite Warming Pesto Lima Beans (pages 148 and 157). It's going to be a delicious chapter!

MY STAPLE INGREDIENTS

To make my weekday suppers even easier, I try to keep my kitchen stocked with a handful of ingredients. You'll find these come up in lots of the recipes, so it's great to have them ready.

Quinoa—comes up a few times in this book. You can keep it for months and won't have to worry about wastage. It is a wonderful source of protein, iron, magnesium and fiber, so it's great for energy. Plus it's easy to digest, is delicious and only takes minutes to cook.

Brown rice—my second favorite grain. As with quinoa, it lasts forever so it's great to stock up on as it can form the basis of so many meals. It does take longer to cook, though, so it's not always as convenient, but if you have that time it's so worth making! It's just as easy to make as white rice, but has so many more vitamins and minerals. The process that produces brown rice removes only the outermost layer of the kernel, so it's far more nutritionally valuable. In contrast, milling white rice actually destroys nearly eighty percent of the vitamins, as well as removing nearly all the fiber and essential fatty acids!

Herbs and spices—a well-stocked herb and spice rack is so important for great savory dishes. In this section you'll find that turmeric, paprika, chili flakes, cumin, ground coriander, dried thyme, dried oregano and dried rosemary are really popular, so I'd recommend stocking up on these. I think it's worth spending a little extra to buy better-quality herbs and spices as they have more flavor, so buy the best you can afford: your meals will taste so much better. And make sure you always have garlic in your fridge.

Condiments—these really bring a recipe to life. The recipes here use a lot of tahini, miso paste, tomato paste, apple cider vinegar, olive oil and raw honey (switch the honey for maple syrup if you prefer, or if you're vegan), so I would recommend stocking up on all these. As with grains and spices, each will last for ages, so while it may be a little expensive the first time you buy your ingredients, each meal will then cost so little that your outlay will even out very quickly.

Canned goods—I find that having cans in my pantry makes life easier. This is especially the case with beans, as you don't have to soak and cook them. Canned black beans, for example, are ready to go instantly, meaning all you have to do is drain, rinse and warm them up, whereas dried beans need to be soaked for six hours or so and then boiled for an hour before you can do anything with them, and sadly I'm not sure most of us have the time or organizational skills to do that! So I stock my pantry with cans of beans, coconut milk and tomatoes.

All the ingredients on the right are used in lots of other recipes in the book, so they'll come in handy at other times, too.

Fresh ingredients—I'm lucky enough to live in the middle of a big city, so I tend to buy most of my fresh produce as and when I need it. But there are a couple of items I buy every week, as I use them so often. I always get potatoes, avocados, spinach and kale, as these come up in at least half my recipes and you can add them to any other dish, too, as they're so versatile: add potatoes to make a recipe more filling, avocados for creaminess and spinach or kale for extra green goodness, for example.

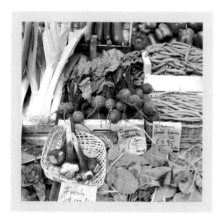

SHOPPING LIST

- APPLE CIDER VINEGAR
- AVOCADOS
- BLACK BEANS
- CHILI FLAKES
- COCONUT MILK
- CORIANDER (GROUND)
- CUCUMBER
- CUMIN (GROUND)
- GARLIC
- HONEY
- KALE
- LEMONS
- MISO PASTE
- MUSTARD SEEDS
- NORI SHEETS
- OLIVE OIL
- PAPRIKA
- PASTA (BROWN RICE)
- POMEGRANATES
- POTATOES
- QUINOA
- RICE (SHORT-GRAIN BROWN)
- SPINACH
- TAHINI
- TAMARI
- THYME, DRIED
- TOMATOES, CANNED
- TOMATO PASTE
- TURMERIC

NOURISHING SOUPS

Warming bowls of goodness to soothe
and nurture your body

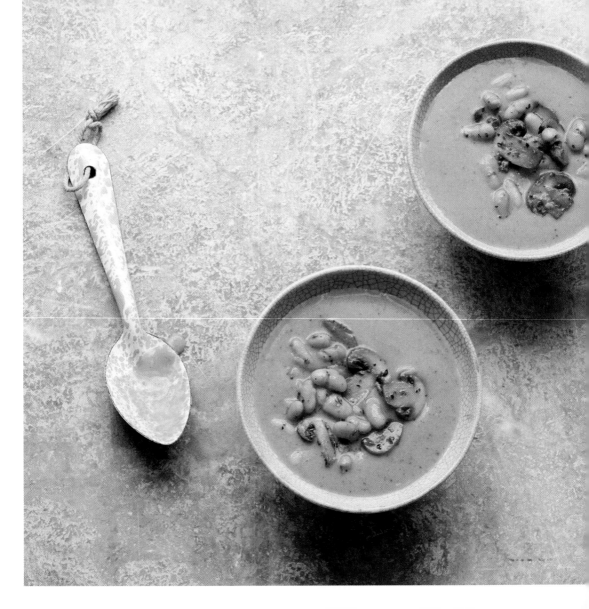

Great if you're in need of an energy boost, as this soup is so full of plant-based protein thanks to the lentils and cannellini beans. Of course it's totally delicious, too, with its warming blend of spices, creamy coconut milk and sweet carrots. I love topping mine with garlic sautéed cannellini beans and mushrooms to give it a heartier texture and make it more filling.

SPICED LENTIL SOUP

Serves 1

For the soup

3 carrots

olive oil

salt and pepper

2 teaspoons mixed herbs (I use herbes de Provence)

1 garlic clove, peeled but whole

2 tablespoons red lentils

½ teaspoon ground turmeric

½ teaspoon ground cumin

½ teaspoon mustard seeds

3 tablespoons coconut milk (ideally, for creaminess), but any plant-based milk will do

For the garlic sautéed beans

¾ cup canned cannellini beans, drained and rinsed

6 cremini mushrooms, finely sliced

1 garlic clove, crushed

2 teaspoons dried mixed herbs

olive oil

salt and pepper

Preheat the oven to 400°F (convection 350°F).

Slice the carrots and place them on a baking sheet with some olive oil, salt and pepper, the mixed herbs and garlic. Bake for 30 minutes, until nice and soft.

Meanwhile, place the lentils in a saucepan of boiling water and boil for about 10 minutes, then reduce the heat and simmer for another 10 minutes, until totally soft. Drain well.

When both the carrots and lentils are cooked, add 1 tablespoon olive oil to a frying pan with the turmeric, cumin and mustard seeds and cook until the mustard seeds start popping. Put the carrots and garlic, lentils, fried spices and coconut milk in a blender, pour in ⅔ cup of water and blend until smooth.

Place the blended soup in a pan to warm gently while you make the topping.

Put the beans and mushrooms in the frying pan in which you fried the spices, adding the crushed garlic, dried herbs and a little olive oil, salt and pepper; using the same pan means that everything will soak up the leftover flavors! Sauté the mixture for 3–4 minutes, until the mushrooms turn slightly brown.

Pour the soup into a bowl and pile the sautéed mushrooms and beans on top.

Tweak It

Use any bean or pulse instead of cannellini, depending on what you prefer or have in the pantry: black beans, white beans and chickpeas all make amazing substitutions.

Probably my favorite soup ever, which is why I've taken it from my blog and shared it with you here. It's so sweet and creamy with subtle hints of coconut, coriander and cumin, plus a hint of chili heat. The color is so beautiful: insanely vibrant and pink, to the point that it's hard to believe it's natural, as it looks more like paint! I love topping my bowl with the roast potato croutons here; they add a whole new level of texture and taste, plus they make it more filling.

BRIGHT PINK SOUP

Serves 1

For the soup

1 small beet
2 medium potatoes
juice of ½ lemon
½ teaspoon chili flakes
½ teaspoon ground cumin
1 garlic clove, crushed
1 teaspoon ground coriander
generous ½ cup coconut milk
salt and pepper

For the croutons

2 medium potatoes
olive oil
1 teaspoon chili flakes
salt and pepper

Preheat the oven to 425°F (convection 400°F). Place the beet, skin on, on a baking sheet and roast for 45 minutes to 1 hour, or until there are bubbles under the skin.

Meanwhile, peel the potatoes for the soup, place them in a saucepan and cover with water. Bring to a boil, then reduce the heat and simmer for about 45 minutes, until really soft.

To make the croutons, chop the potatoes (no need to peel) into small, bite-size pieces and place them on a baking sheet with lots of olive oil plus the chili flakes, salt and pepper. Bake for 45 minutes, until crispy outside and tender within.

When the beet is cool enough to handle, peel. Chop it in half and place it in a blender. Drain the boiled (soup) potatoes and add them to the blender with the lemon juice, chili flakes, cumin, garlic, coriander and coconut milk, plus some salt and pepper. Blend until smooth; if you find it's too thick, add water until you reach your desired consistency.

Place in a saucepan and heat it up to the perfect temperature. Pour into a bowl and sprinkle with the roast potato croutons.

Kitchen Know-How

Save time by using ready-cooked beet, just be sure to check there aren't any additives in it.

Tweak It

These croutons go well with many of my other soups, so go ahead and experiment.

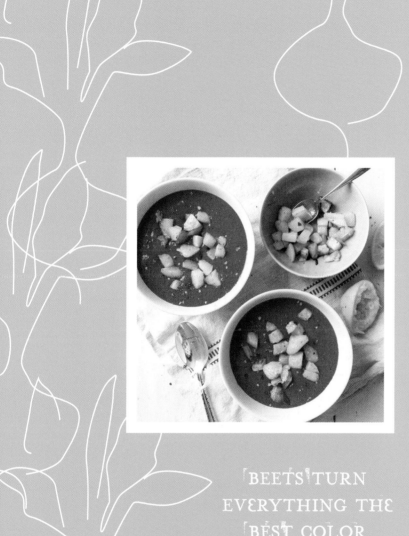

BEETS TURN
EVERYTHING THE
BEST COLOR

Sweet potato wedges with cinnamon and paprika have been one of my favorite foods for years, so I decided to try to turn the winning combination into a soup. I added a little coconut milk to make it extra creamy, tamari and mustard seeds for a rich taste and apple cider vinegar for a tang . . . and the result was a success.

SWEET POTATO AND COCONUT SOUP

Serves 2

2 sweet potatoes
one 14-ounce can coconut milk
¼ cup cilantro leaves
2 teaspoons tamari
2 teaspoons paprika
2 teaspoons ground cinnamon
I teaspoon apple cider vinegar
I teaspoon mustard seeds

Peel the sweet potatoes, chop them into bite-size chunks and place them in a steamer. Steam them for about 45 minutes, until they're really soft.

Put the sweet potatoes in a blender with all the remaining ingredients. Pour in ¾ cup of water and blend until smooth.

Transfer the soup to a saucepan and heat gently until it's nice and warm.

Make It Better

Try dipping sweet potato wedges (page 187) into the soup instead of bread, for extra sweet potato goodness!

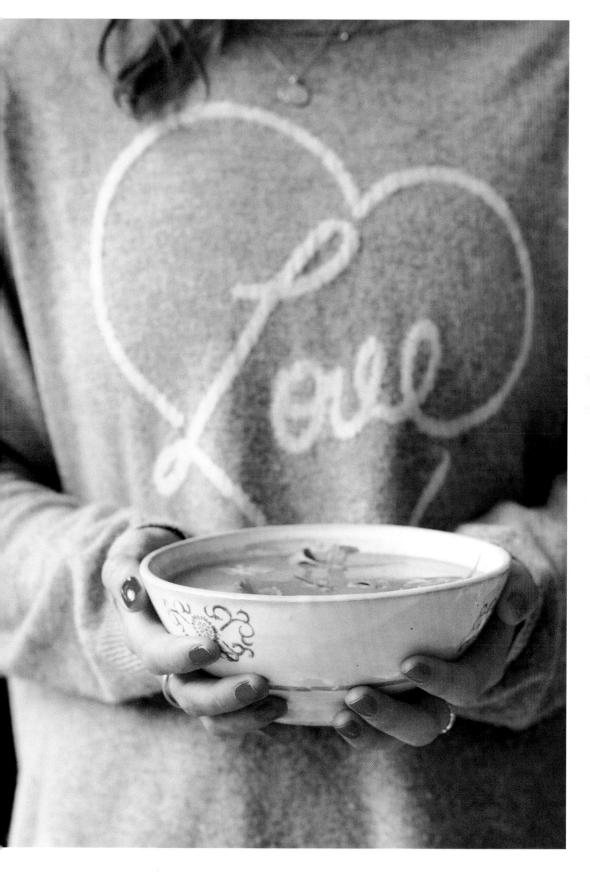

My favorite soup to make in big batches, as it's so easy to put together, which is why I've designed the recipe to serve four, so you can portion up servings and freeze them to save for later. It is so easy to adapt, too; I use the recipe below as my base and then throw any leftover veggies into it to stop them from going to waste.

CLEAN-OUT-THE-FRIDGE SOUP

Serves 4

1 beet
4 carrots
4 parsnips
olive oil
salt and pepper
3 teaspoons miso paste
3 teaspoons apple cider vinegar
2 teaspoons ground cumin

Preheat the oven to 350°F (convection 325°F).

Place the whole beet on a baking sheet (don't worry about taking off the skin) and cook for about 1 hour.

Peel and chop the carrots and parsnips and add to the baking sheet after 20 minutes, so they cook for 40 minutes, drizzling everything with olive oil and seasoning with salt and pepper.

Once the roots have cooked, peel the beet, then add it to a blender with the carrots, parsnips, miso, vinegar, salt, pepper, cumin and 6 cups of water. Blend until smooth. Reheat gently to serve.

Make it Better

If you're feeling hungrier than soup, but already have some of this in your freezer, try stirring sautéed mushrooms and buckwheat noodles into your bowl for a heartier meal.

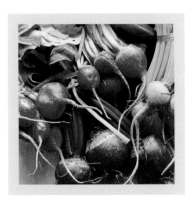

A great dinner option if you're not that hungry as, despite feeling very comforting, it's pretty light. I add sautéed kale to the soup at the last minute, to lend a more interesting texture and give a good dose of greens to keep you feeling awesome. It is also a great starter if you're having a dinner party, as it means people will still be hungry for the main course.

CHUNKY CARROT AND KALE SOUP

Serves 2

3 carrots
1 parsnip
2 red bell peppers
olive oil
salt and pepper
one 15-ounce can cannellini
    beans, drained and rinsed
1 tablespoon apple cider vinegar
½–1 teaspoon chili flakes
1 teaspoon ground cumin
1 teaspoon ground ginger
1 teaspoon paprika
1 teaspoon tamari
4 ounces kale
2 garlic cloves, crushed

Preheat the oven to 350°F (convection 325°F).

Chop the carrots, parsnip and bell peppers into chunks, place them on a baking sheet, drizzle with olive oil and season with salt and pepper. Place in the oven and cook for 45 minutes, giving them a shake halfway through.

Add the roasted veggies to a food processor with all the remaining ingredients, except the kale and garlic. Pour in 2½ cups of water and blend until the soup is still a bit chunky. (You may need to blend in batches.)

While this happens, tear the kale leaves from the stems and put the leaves into a frying pan with a little olive oil and the garlic. Lightly sauté the kale for a few minutes until it softens and the garlic has turned translucent.

Once the kale is soft, add it to a saucepan along with the soup and warm them both up together until they're nice and hot.

Tweak It

If you want to make this richer and heavier, blend another can of cannellini beans into the mixture, or a couple of boiled potatoes. This makes it creamier, too!

I never used to like cold soups, but last summer I got so into them and this was one of my favorites. The blend of avocado, cucumber, cashew milk, lime juice and spices makes such a creamy, refreshing bowlful. The perfect meal for an easy warm-weather supper, as all you have to do is blend the ingredients together to create something amazing. I love serving this with a big handful of seeds sprinkled over, to add a great crunch.

CLEANSING AVOCADO AND CUCUMBER SOUP

Serves 2

1 avocado (7 ounces, unpeeled weight)
⅓ cucumber (4 ounces), plus more if needed
scant ½ cup cashew milk (or any plant-based milk, just make sure it's not sweetened)
juice of 1 lime
1 tablespoon tahini
1 teaspoon honey
1 teaspoon dried oregano
½ teaspoon chili flakes, plus more to serve (optional)
1 teaspoon ground coriander
1 garlic clove, crushed
salt and lots of pepper
handful of sunflower and pumpkin seeds, to serve (optional)

Scoop the avocado flesh out of the skin and into a blender. Cut the cucumber into chunks, leaving the skin on. If the cucumber has a lot of large seeds in it, then discard these and add extra cucumber to make its weight up to 4 ounces. Add to the blender.

Add all the remaining ingredients, except the seeds, to the blender, pour in a scant ½ cup of water and blend until smooth and creamy, this should take a minute or so.

Pour the soup into bowls and serve straight away. I like sprinkling chili flakes and a handful of a pumpkin and sunflowers seeds over the top; they make it look beautiful and the seeds add a delicious crunch, as well as a protein boost. Store in the fridge, so it can be served chilled.

Tweak It

This works well warm, too, so if you're not a cold soup fan you can try gently heating it; but don't let it boil, as it can become a little lumpy.

Kitchen Know-How

You can take this soup out with you; just pour it into an airtight glass jar, as you would a smoothie.

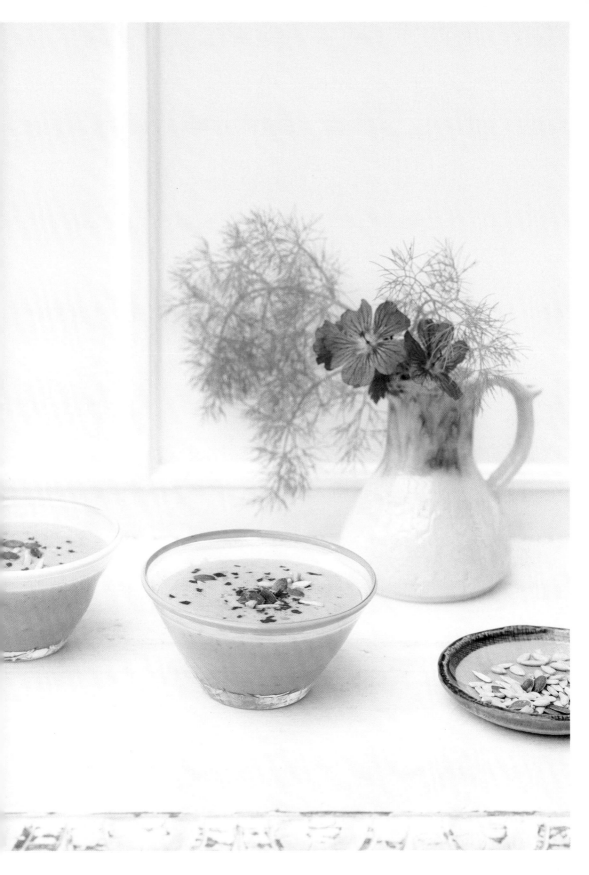

EASY
VEGGIES

Bowls of comfort and happiness

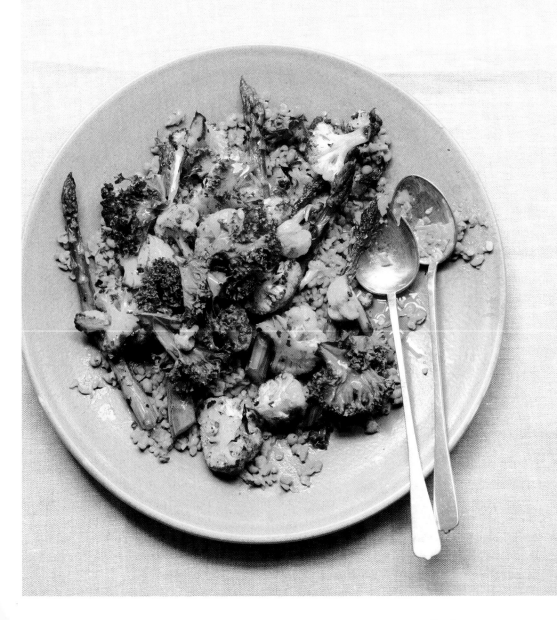

This is one of my favorite weekday suppers, it feels so nourishing and comforting but it's nice and light at the same time. It also contains four portions of veggies, which is awesome, especially if you feel you've been lacking goodness in your other meals. The lime-infused pea mash goes so well with the chili and turmeric cauliflower.

PEA AND CAULIFLOWER BOWL

 Serves 1

⅓ head of cauliflower
⅓ teaspoon ground turmeric
½ teaspoon chili flakes
salt and pepper
olive oil
handful of asparagus
    (about 8 spears)
3 big handfuls of kale
    (about 3 ounces)
1½ cups frozen peas
juice of 1½ limes

Preheat the oven to 400°F (convection 350°F).

Chop the cauliflower into florets and place these on a large baking sheet (with space for the asparagus and kale) with the turmeric, chili flakes, lots of pepper, a little salt and a drizzling of olive oil. Put in the oven to cook for 25 minutes.

After 10 minutes, add the asparagus to the baking sheet.

Finally, 5–8 minutes before the end, put the torn-up kale leaves on the baking sheet, too (discard the stems and ribs), with an extra sprinkling of salt.

Meanwhile, put the peas in a saucepan of cold water and bring them to a boil, allowing them to cook for 10 minutes. Drain them and place in a bowl with pepper, salt, the lime juice and 1 tablespoon of olive oil, then mash the peas.

Arrange the baked veggies on the bed of pea mash to serve.

Shop Sense

To avoid wastage, roast the whole head of the cauliflower and all the asparagus in the bunch and store the leftovers in the fridge. Roast veg makes a great addition to any meal!

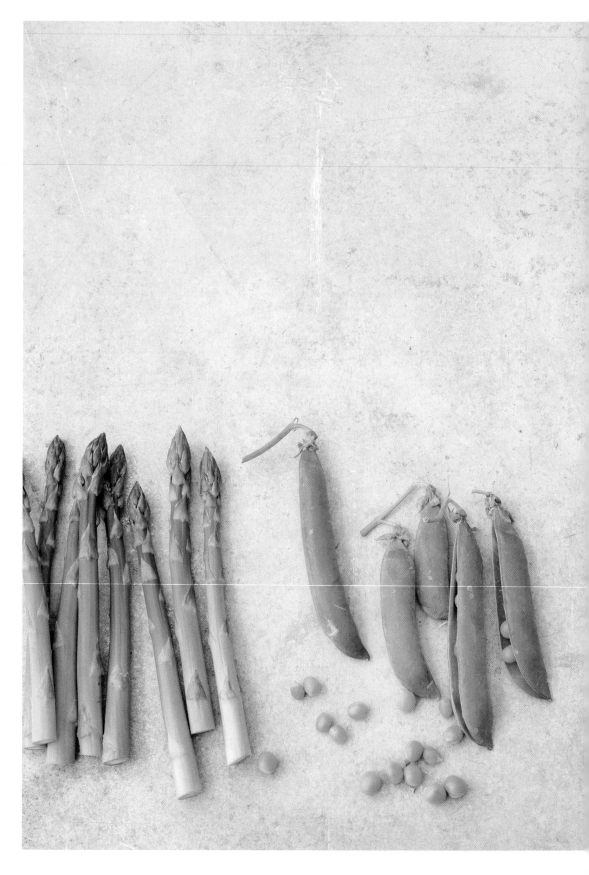

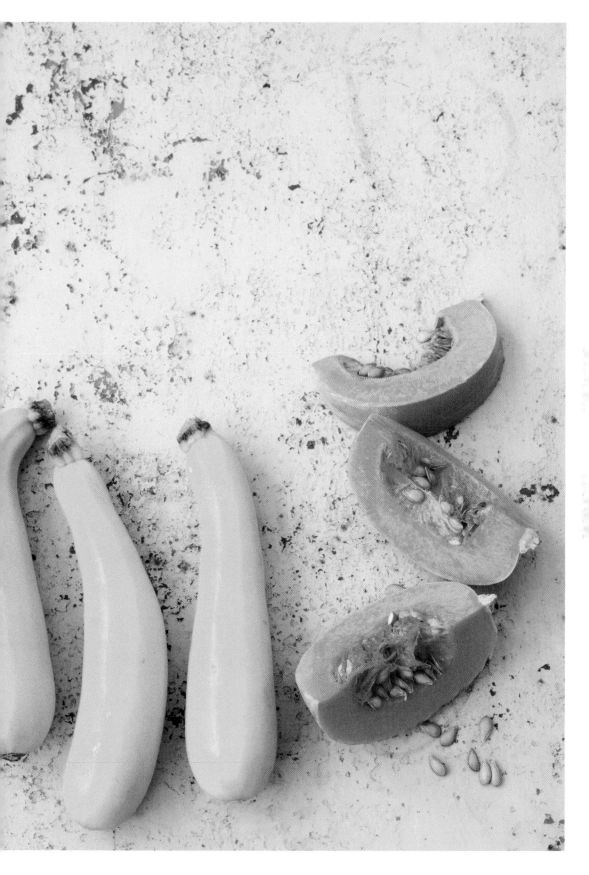

The perfect weeknight dinner, filling and delicious yet so energizing and nourishing. It's easy to throw together, too. I make big batches of brown rice every weekend so that I can put the whole thing together in just twenty minutes. My favorite thing about this recipe is the way that all the ingredients complement each other, from the slightly firm eggplant slices to the soft wilted spinach, the garlic sautéed black beans, the toasted sunflower seeds and the warming brown rice, all mixed with rich tahini, salty tamari and tangy lemon juice to create lots of incredible flavor and a creamy texture.

ROASTED EGGPLANT AND TAHINI BOWL

Serves 1

½ cup brown rice
2 teaspoons tamari
1 eggplant
olive oil
salt and pepper
3.5 ounces spinach
1 garlic clove, crushed
2 heaping tablespoons tahini,
    plus more to serve
¾ cup canned black beans,
    drained and rinsed
juice of 1 lemon
big handful of sunflower and
    pumpkin seeds

Start by placing the brown rice in a saucepan with 2 cups of boiling water and 1 teaspoon of the tamari. Allow it to simmer for about 40 minutes until cooked; make sure that it never runs out of water.

Once the rice has been cooking for 15 minutes or so, preheat the oven to 400°F (convection 350°F). Then cut the eggplant into very thin slices, about ⅛ inch thick.

Oil a baking sheet with olive oil and place the eggplant slices on it, then drizzle a little more olive oil on them plus some salt and pepper. Put the baking sheet into the oven for 15–20 minutes until they are starting to go crispy, but not burnt.

Next, sauté the spinach: simply place it in a frying pan with a little olive oil, the garlic, salt, pepper and half the tahini. Allow it to wilt for a few minutes.

Once the spinach has cooked, add the beans. Sauté for a couple more minutes until they are warm and delicious.

When the rice finishes cooking, stir in the second tablespoon of tahini, the second teaspoon of tamari and the lemon juice.

Finally, toast the sunflower and pumpkin seeds for 1 minute or so in a dry frying pan.

Then place everything together in a bowl, drizzling with extra tahini, before enjoying.

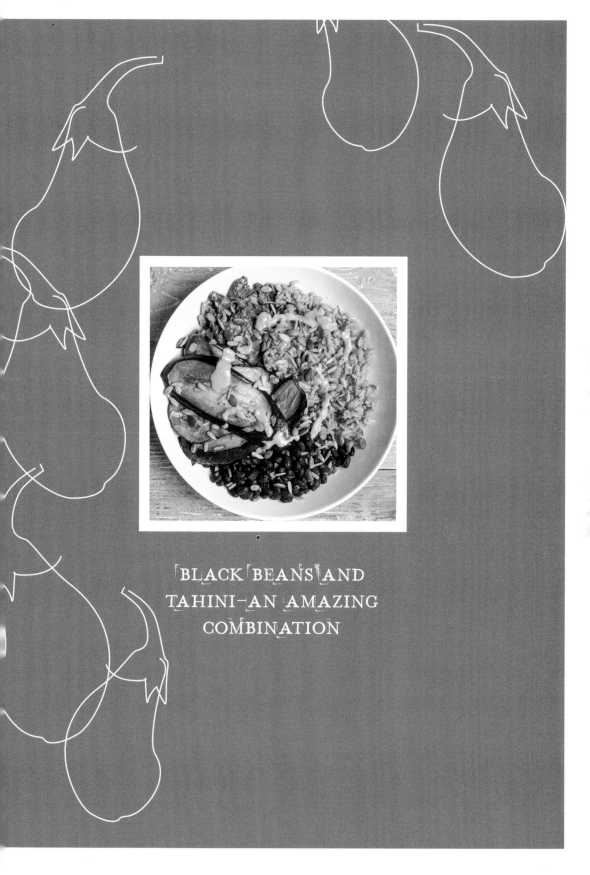

BLACK BEANS AND TAHINI-AN AMAZING COMBINATION

I've always been resistant to stuffed peppers, as they were so stereotypical of mediocre vegetarian food, but recently I've been experimenting a lot with them and have realized that they're the best, easy dinner for one and that I shouldn't have ruled them out for so long! This fuss-free recipe really fills you up and leaves you feeling satisfied with minimal effort. I love serving the pepper on a bed of sautéed garlicky spinach or an arugula salad, as the colors look so pretty.

MUSHROOM-STUFFED PEPPERS

Serves 1

1 red bell pepper
olive oil
2 tablespoons pine nuts
2 garlic cloves, crushed
6 cremini mushrooms,
    roughly chopped
salt and pepper
juice of ½ lime
1 teaspoon tahini

Preheat the oven to 350°F (convection 325°F).

Halve the bell pepper lengthwise (through the stem). Cut out and discard the middle, seedy part. Put the halves on a baking sheet, then drizzle with olive oil and bake for 10 minutes.

Meanwhile, place a dry frying pan over medium heat and toast the pine nuts until they start to turn golden and release a little bit of oil. Tip them into a bowl.

Using the same pan, drizzle in a little olive oil and add the garlic, mushrooms and a little salt and pepper. Sauté the mushrooms for about 5 minutes until they're nice and soft.

Once they're cooked, mix the mushrooms with the pine nuts, lime juice and tahini, then season with salt and pepper.

Take the bell pepper halves out the oven and stuff them with the mushroom mixture, then put them back in the oven to bake for another 15 minutes.

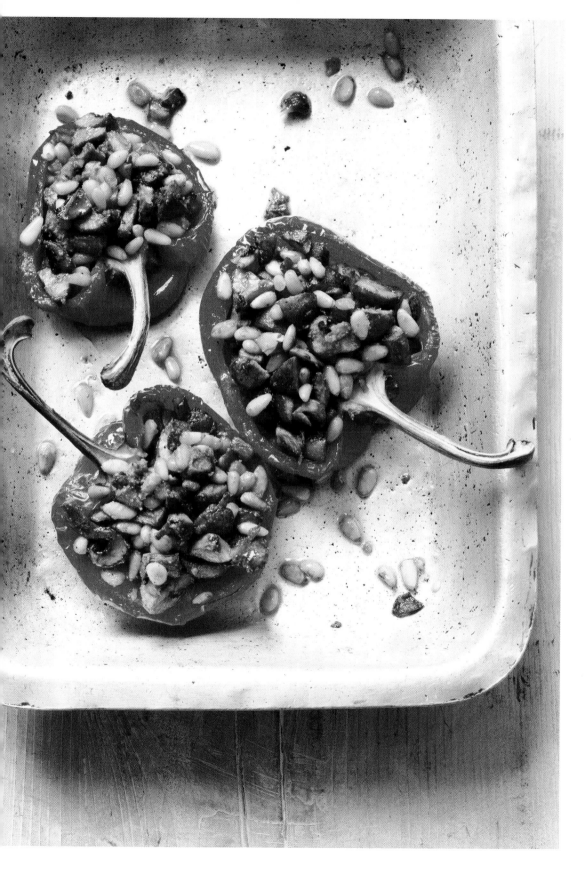

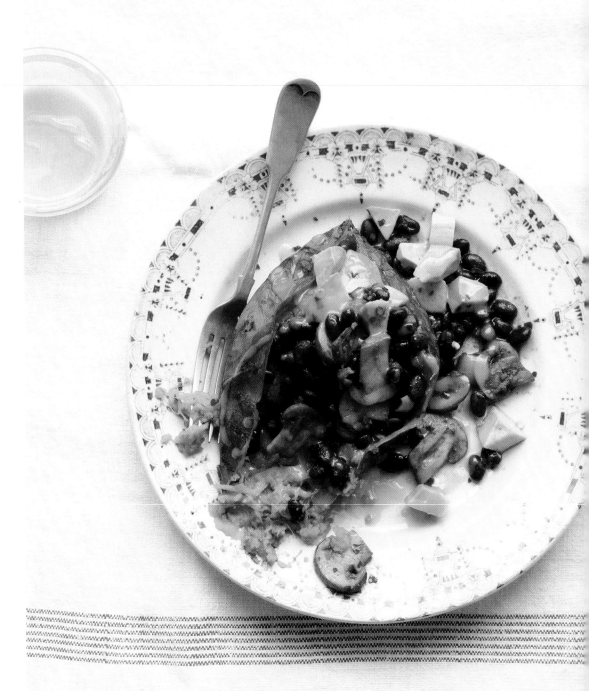

Sweet potatoes are one of my absolute favorite foods. I love regular potatoes but I find that, on their own, sweet potatoes have more flavor, so I prefer baking these. All baked sweet potatoes are great, but this filling makes them extra-specially good! I sauté a topping of mushrooms and black beans with crushed garlic, chili flakes, ground coriander and pepper before drizzling a sweet tahini dressing all over everything: so amazing!

THE BEST BAKED SWEET POTATO

Serves 1

For the sweet potato

1 medium-small sweet potato
7 mushrooms, finely sliced
¾ cup canned black beans, drained and rinsed
3 garlic cloves, crushed
1 teaspoon chili flakes
1 teaspoon ground coriander
salt and pepper
olive oil
1 small avocado

For the dressing

2 teaspoons tahini
juice of 1 lime
1 teaspoon honey
2 teaspoons olive oil

Preheat the oven to 425°F (convection 400°F).

Prick the sweet potato several times with a fork (this lets the steam escape and stops it from exploding in the oven), wrap it in foil, then place it on a baking sheet and let it bake for about 1 hour, or until tender.

Meanwhile, prepare everything else. Place the mushrooms in a frying pan with the beans, garlic, chili flakes, coriander, salt, pepper and lots of olive oil. Sauté for 5–8 minutes, until the mushrooms are nice and soft.

Make the dressing. Combine all the ingredients in a mug with 2 teaspoons of water, then whisk them with a little salt.

Once the potato has cooked, slice it almost in half and fill it with the mushroom mixture, the avocado—chopped—and the tahini dressing.

Tweak It

If you don't have any black beans, try using cannellini beans, or experiment with a mix of the two.

HEARTY
GRAINS
AND BEANS

Sustaining, super-filling recipes to fuel your day

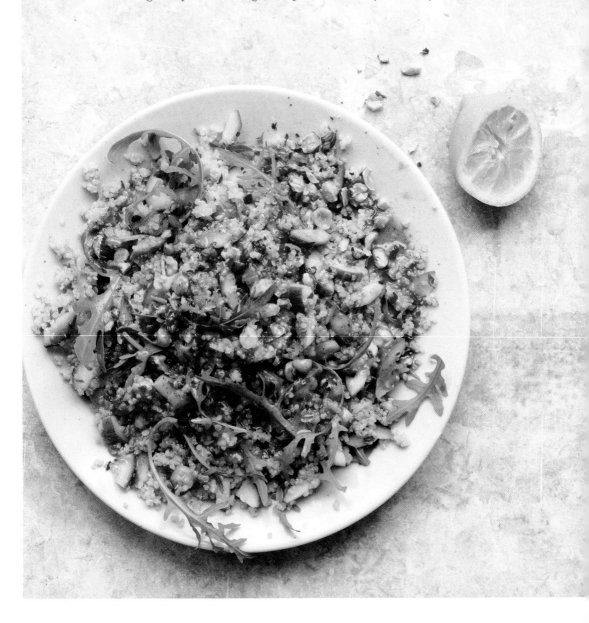

My favorite post-yoga or -gym dinner, quick to make and so energizing after a big workout. The mix of quinoa, almond butter and hazelnuts is really filling, so you'll feel replenished and satisfied by the time you finish your bowl. I should warn you though: the dressing is so addictive . . . if you're anything like me, you'll have eaten it all before the quinoa has even cooked, so be prepared to make two batches of it!

ALMOND BUTTER QUINOA

Serves 1

For the quinoa

⅓ cup quinoa
juice of ½ lemon
salt
handful of hazelnuts (1.5 ounces)
½ small cucumber
big handful of arugula

For the dressing

2 tablespoons almond butter
2 tablespoons olive oil
juice of ½ lemon
½ teaspoon chili flakes

Preheat the oven to 425°F (convection 400°F).

Place the quinoa in a saucepan with a generous 1 cup of boiling water, the lemon juice and a little salt. Let it boil for a minute or so, then reduce the heat, place the lid on the pan and let it simmer for another 10–15 minutes, until all the water has been absorbed and the quinoa is fluffy but not mushy.

Meanwhile, put the hazelnuts on a baking sheet and let them bake for about 10 minutes until they're crunchy (keep an eye on them so that they don't burn).

Slice the cucumber lengthwise into quarters, then into eighths. Discard the seedy central part and then slice into thin pieces.

Mix the dressing ingredients in a mug, adding 2 tablespoons of water and a little salt.

Once the quinoa has cooked, place it in a bowl with the hazelnuts, cucumber and arugula, then pour the dressing on top and mix it all together.

Kitchen Know-How

Use this dressing for any grains, it instantly adds a creamy texture and rich flavor that livens up any dish.

If you're feeling in need of vitamins, minerals and general health-giving food, then this is for you. It will instantly make you feel amazing and the four varieties of greens will revive your body. It's a very simple dish that's easy on the digestion, too; so if you haven't been that kind to your stomach for a few days, it will do wonders to restore the balance. It's delicious, thanks to the creamy tahini and garlic dressing, which I like to generously pour over everything!

GREEN GOODNESS BOWL

Serves 1

For the bowl

⅓ cup quinoa
juice of ½ lemon
salt
1 small zucchini
olive oil
5 spears broccolini
big handful of kale
big handful of spinach

For the dressing

1 tablespoon tahini
1 tablespoon olive oil
1 teaspoon miso paste
juice of 1 lemon
2 garlic cloves, crushed
½ teaspoon cayenne pepper

Place the quinoa in a saucepan with a generous 1 cup of boiling water, the lemon juice and a little salt. Let it boil for a minute or so, then reduce the heat, place the lid on the pan and let it simmer for another 10–15 minutes, until all the water has been absorbed and the quinoa is fluffy but not mushy.

Slice the zucchini in half, then cut it into thin half-moon shapes. Place these in a frying pan with a little olive oil and salt and sauté them for a couple of minutes over low heat.

Meanwhile, steam the broccolini, kale and spinach. The broccolini will take a few minutes longer to cook, so put that in before the others.

Mix all the dressing ingredients together in a mug, adding 1 tablespoon of water.

Once everything has cooked, assemble it in a bowl. I like to put the quinoa on one side and the veg on another, before pouring the dressing over everything.

Tweak It

This works with any grain so if you have some brown rice or buckwheat that's ready to go use that instead of quinoa.

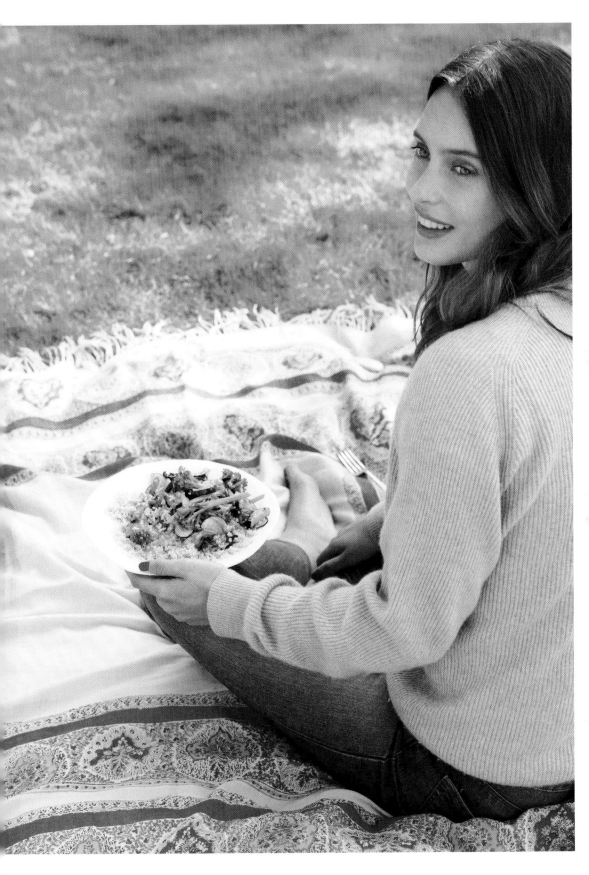

Most of my girlfriends would say this is their favorite dish in the book; they're all obsessed with it! They all adore it served with a simple arugula salad and lots of creamy Sweet Potato and Garlic Purée (page 65); it's such a great dinner! The honey and apple cider vinegar dressing does wonders for the dish; it makes it so wonderfully sweet and contrasts perfectly with the mushroom and spinach mix.

HONEY AND MUSHROOM QUINOA

Serves 2

For the quinoa

⅔ cup quinoa

1½ tablespoons tamari

1 large beet

12 mushrooms

2 garlic cloves, crushed

1 teaspoon ground turmeric

1 teaspoon chili powder

¼ cup olive oil

¼ cup apple cider vinegar

3.5 ounces spinach

For the dressing

3 tablespoons olive oil

1 tablespoon apple cider vinegar

2 tablespoons honey

½ teaspoon ground turmeric

Place the quinoa in a pan with 2 cups water and 1 tablespoon of the tamari. Let this cook for 12–15 minutes.

Meanwhile, peel the beet, then grate it using the fine side of a grater. Cut the mushrooms into thin slices.

Place the crushed garlic, turmeric and chili powder into a saucepan with the olive oil. Let this cook for a minute or so until the spices are bubbling nicely, being careful not to brown the garlic. Add the mushrooms and beet with the remaining ½ tablespoon of tamari and the vinegar, then let them cook until the mushrooms are soft. Stir in the spinach.

Mix all the ingredients for the dressing together.

Once the quinoa has cooked, mix it with the vegetables before pouring the dressing over everything.

One of my favorite weekday dinners: simple and comforting. It's not as fancy as some of the other recipes in this chapter—more kitchen supper than dinner party—but I could eat bowls and bowls of it. The potatoes and lentils together are so hearty and satisfying, while the tomato, garlic and herbs create the best sauce, bursting with flavor in each mouthful. Just don't try serving this to someone who doesn't like lentils, as it's very lentil-heavy so there's no hiding from them!

HERBED LENTIL BOWL

Serves 4

scant ½ cup Puy lentils

one 14.5-ounce can diced tomatoes

2 tablespoons tomato paste

2 teaspoons dried thyme

2 teaspoons dried oregano

2 teaspoons dried rosemary

2 garlic cloves, crushed

12 cherry tomatoes

15 baby potatoes (10 ounces)

1 carrot

juice of ½ lemon

Place the lentils in a large saucepan with the canned tomatoes, tomato paste, dried herbs and garlic, then stir in 2½ cups of water. Place the lid on the pan and bring it all to a boil, then reduce the heat to a simmer.

Chop the cherry tomatoes into quarters and add these to the lentil mixture.

Halve the potatoes and add these to the pan. Cook for about 50 minutes, or until the liquid has been absorbed and the potatoes are soft.

Meanwhile, peel and grate the carrot. Once the lentils have cooked for about 25 minutes, stir in the grated carrot.

When everything is cooked, stir in the lemon juice and let it all cook together for 1 minute or so, then serve.

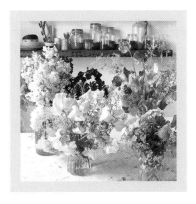

This recipe is for my sisters, who are mashed potato addicts! If you ask them what they want for dinner, they almost always say "mash," so I got more inventive with the mash to keep it interesting. Keeping the skin on the potato adds great texture, while the mustard seeds, cumin and chili flakes create a delicious, rich flavor. It is rougher than conventional mash, which I love, especially with the sautéed veggies and crispy kale. If you're after a comforting meal that boosts your greens intake, you need this!

COMFORTING MASHED POTATO BOWL

Serves 1

2 medium potatoes (10 ounces total)
6 baby corns
½ zucchini
3 spears broccolini
¼ cup olive oil, plus more for drizzling
salt and pepper
1 teaspoon dried thyme
big handful of kale
1 teaspoon ground cumin
½ teaspoon mustard seeds
½ teaspoon chili flakes

Cut the potatoes into quarters; no need to peel them here. Place them in a saucepan, cover them with cold water and bring to a boil, then reduce the heat to a simmer and cook for 25–30 minutes, or until they're really nice and soft.

Meanwhile, prepare the rest of the veg. Cut the corns in half lengthwise and slice the zucchini into rounds. Cut the broccolini stalks into 1-inch-long sticks and the heads in half.

Preheat the oven to 400°F (convection 350°F).

Put the broccolini stalks into a frying pan with with the ¼ cup olive oil, salt and pepper and cook for about 5 minutes, then add the corn, zucchini, broccolini heads and thyme. Cook for 15 minutes, tossing every few minutes so it doesn't burn.

Tear the kale from the stems and place the leaves on a baking sheet with a drizzle of olive oil and salt. Place in the oven and cook for about 8 minutes, so the kale is crispy but not burnt.

Once the potatoes have finished cooking, drain and place in a bowl. Mash them roughly with a fork, pour in a drizzle of olive oil and add the cumin, mustard seeds and chili flakes, plus salt and pepper. Mix together, then put the potato in a bowl and pile the sautéed veg and crispy kale on top.

Make It Better

Be patient with the potatoes, it's so important to wait until they're really soft before mashing them, otherwise you'll have lumpy mash.

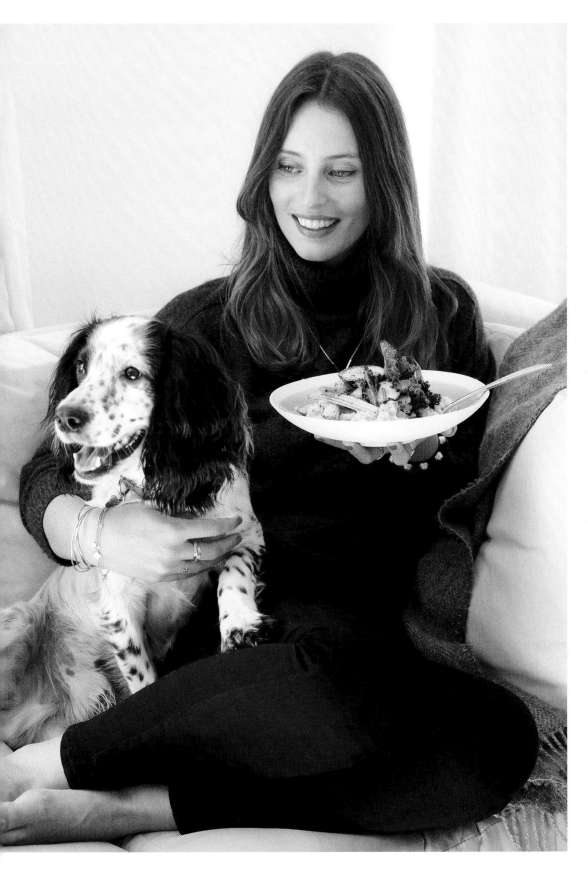

I've always adored tomato pasta. It's such a simple dish that, when done right, tastes better than almost anything else. For me it's the ultimate comfort food, especially at the end of a long day when the weather is cold and I need something warming. This recipe takes just ten minutes from start to finish and the only fresh ingredients you need are tomatoes, so it's about as easy as it gets! Plus there's almost no chopping involved, which is perfect if you're tired.

EASY PASTA ARRABBIATA

Serves 1

I serving of pasta (I use 3.5 ounces brown rice pasta)
I heaping teaspoon dried oregano
I heaping teaspoon dried thyme
I heaping teaspoon chili flakes
2 garlic cloves, crushed
2 tablespoons olive oil
I2 cherry tomatoes
half a 14.5-ounce can diced tomatoes
I tablespoon tomato paste
juice of ½ lemon
salt and pepper

Put the pasta on to cook, according to the package instructions.

Meanwhile, put the dried oregano, thyme, chili flakes and garlic into a frying pan with the olive oil. Let these cook while you cut the cherry tomatoes into quarters.

Add the tomatoes to the frying pan with the canned tomatoes and tomato paste. Let this cook for about 5 minutes, until the cherry tomatoes are nice and soft. Add the lemon juice and season with salt and pepper.

Once the pasta has cooked, drain it, then stir it into the sauce.

Tweak It

To twiddle this up, try adding sautéed mushrooms and spinach; the veggies add more flavors and textures.

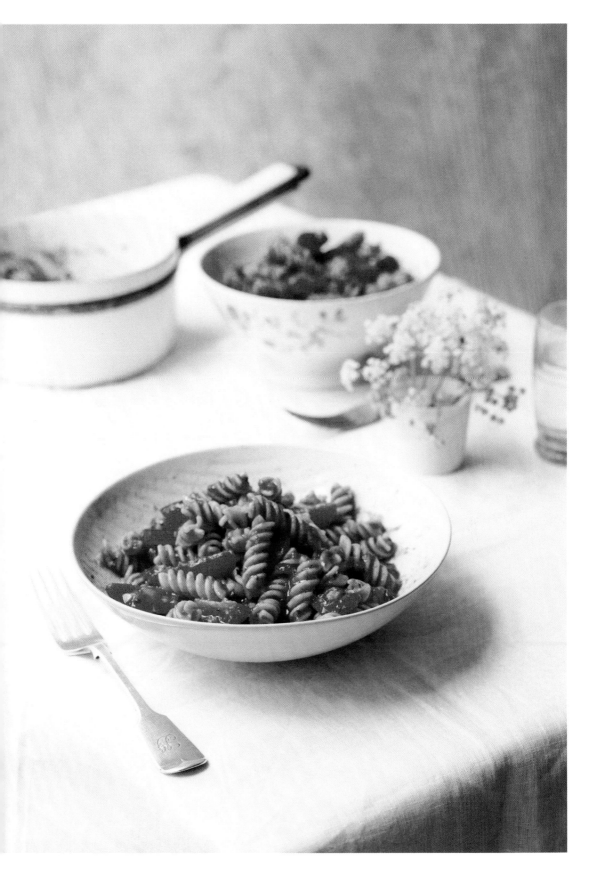

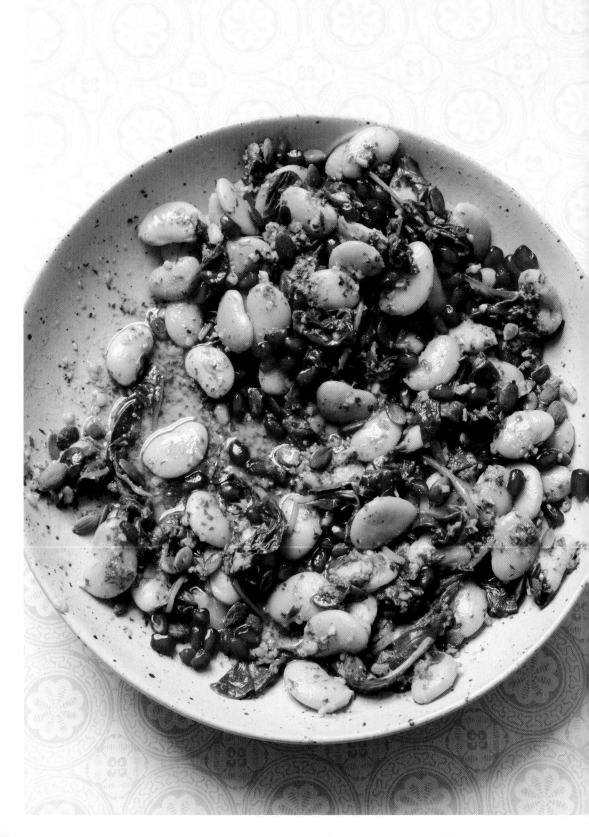

A favorite recipe from my blog, which I hope you'll love. It's incredibly simple but very addictive; the first time I made this I cooked it four or five times in the following two weeks! There's just something about the mix of soft, buttery beans smothered in homemade pesto with sautéed spinach, crunchy pumpkin seeds and sweet, juicy pomegranates that I can't get enough of.

WARMING PESTO LIMA BEANS

Serves 1

For the pesto

1 garlic clove
6 tablespoons pine nuts
big handful of fresh basil
    leaves (1 ounce)
3 tablespoons olive oil
juice of 1 lemon
salt and pepper

For the salad

one 15-ounce can lima beans,
    drained and rinsed
3.5 ounces spinach
olive oil
juice of 1 lemon
pepper
handful of pumpkin seeds
sprinkling of pomegranate
    seeds

Start by making the pesto. Simply peel the garlic and then put all the ingredients into a food processor and blend until smooth. Set aside.

Place the beans in a frying pan with the spinach and pesto and sauté everything in a splash of olive oil for 2–3 minutes until the spinach has wilted and everything is warm.

While they cook, squeeze the lemon (for the salad) over the beans and add pepper.

Place the pesto beans and spinach into a bowl and sprinkle the pumpkin and pomegranate seeds over the top.

Tweak It

In hot weather, swap the wilted spinach for fresh arugula and serve this as a cold salad.

One of the first recipes I ever put on my blog, which makes it quite special! I still love it though and make it a lot for easy weekday suppers both for myself and when I have a couple of friends over. It's a fun recipe to make as you have to really get involved with your hands. You can add any veggies to the inside of your roll, my staples are carrot, zucchini and red pepper but broccoli, cauliflower, cucumber and asparagus are all awesome, too.

QUINOA NORI ROLLS WITH AVOCADO CREAM

Serves 1

For the rolls

2½ tablespoons quinoa
juice of 1 lemon
1 carrot
1 zucchini
1 red bell pepper
handful of sesame seeds
2–3 nori sheets

For the avocado cream

1 avocado
1 tablespoon apple cider vinegar
1 tablespoon olive oil
juice of 1 lime
salt

Start by cooking the quinoa. Place it in a small saucepan with ½ cup of water and the lemon juice. Bring to a boil, then reduce the heat and simmer for 10–15 minutes, until all the water has been absorbed and the quinoa is fluffy but not mushy.

Meanwhile, chop all the veggies into thin, long strips.

Now make the avocado cream. Simply scoop the avocado flesh out of its skin and into a food processor with all the other ingredients and 1 tablespoon of water. Blend for a few minutes until a creamy paste forms.

Once the quinoa has cooked, let it cool for a few minutes, then stir in the sesame seeds.

Next assemble your rolls. The best way to do this is to lay a nori sheet on a work surface, put a layer of avocado cream in a strip on one long side, then top it with a sprinkling of quinoa and veggies. Once you're ready, roll it up tightly. Repeat to fill and roll the other nori sheets.

Either eat the rolls whole, or chop them into bite-size pieces with a sharp, preferably serrated knife.

Tweak It

For a protein boost, add bean sprouts, pumpkin seeds or black beans to your roll; they all add great flavor and texture, too.

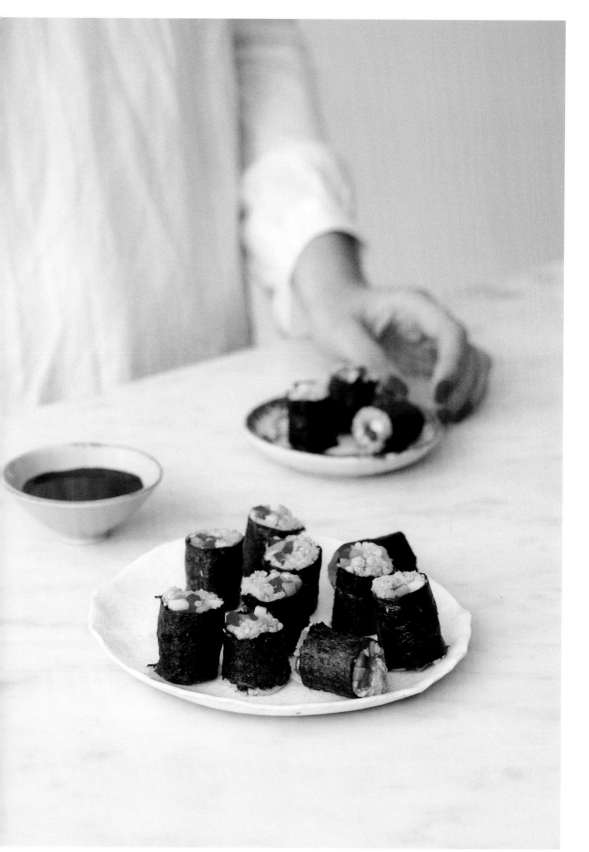

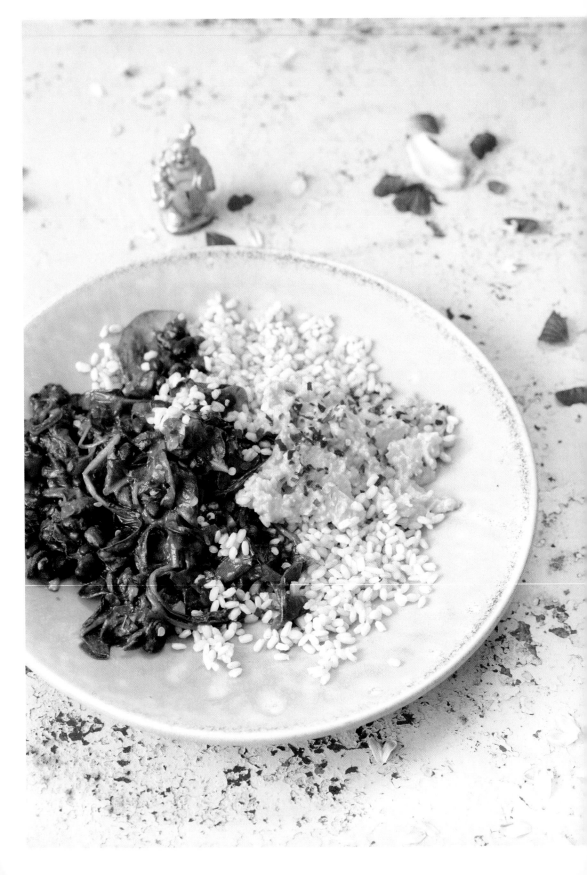

I ate this meal almost every night for a few months last year, I just couldn't get enough of it! I'd make a big batch of brown rice on the weekend so that the whole thing would take just five minutes to prepare, making it the perfect supper for those evenings when you come home starving and need something delicious very quickly! The rich miso, chili and garlic really bring the other ingredients to life.

BUDDHA BOWL

Serves 1

⅓ cup short-grain brown rice

5 ounces spinach

½ cup canned black beans, drained and rinsed

2 garlic cloves, crushed

2 teaspoons tomato paste

2 teaspoons miso paste

olive oil

salt and pepper

½ avocado

chili flakes

Place the brown rice in a saucepan with a generous ¾ cup of boiling water and let this simmer for 35–40 minutes, until the rice is soft and the water has been absorbed.

Place the spinach in a frying pan with the beans, garlic, tomato paste, miso, a little olive oil, salt and pepper. Gently heat this for about 5 minutes, until the spinach has wilted.

Mash the avocado with a sprinkling of chili flakes.

Finally, place everything together in a shallow bowl.

BIG-BATCH COOKING

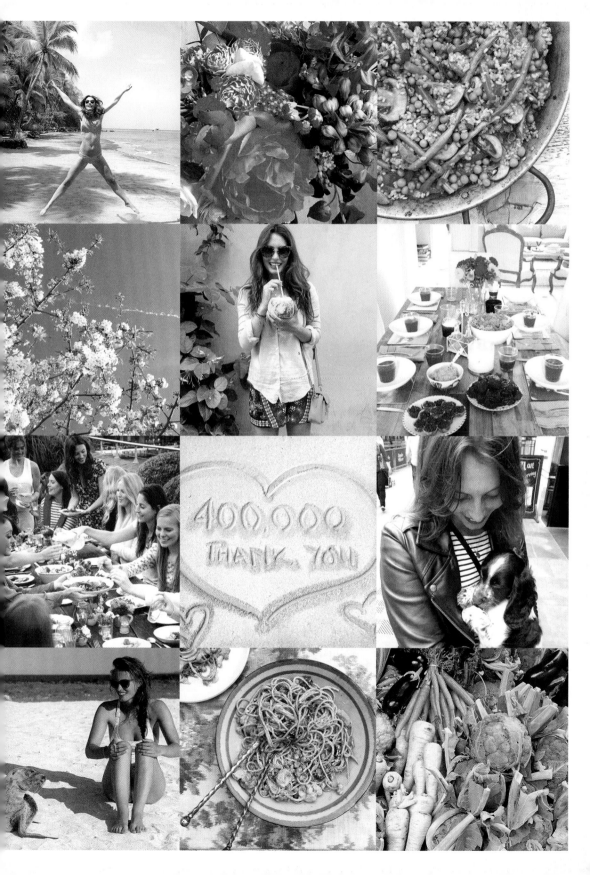

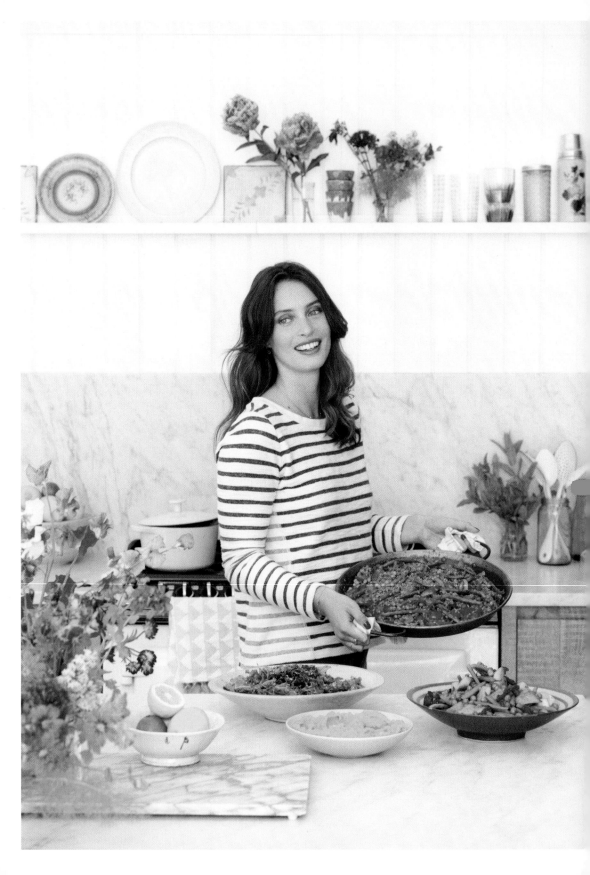

BIG-BATCH COOKING

I absolutely love hosting dinner parties, as they combine all my favorite things: cooking, eating, hanging out with the people I love and being cozy at home. I really enjoy decorating the table with beautiful crockery, flowers and tea lights; piling big bowls high with delicious-smelling food and then watching everyone tuck in and enjoy themselves. The only hard part is deciding what to make, especially when everyone has different eating habits and you're pressed for time . . . which is where these recipes come in!

The dishes in this chapter have been designed to feed lots of people with minimal effort, not because you don't love your friends and family, but because I appreciate that it's rare for most people to have hours of spare time, and, even if you do, that you may not want to spend it chopping and cooking.

I make this food for easy kitchen suppers with girlfriends, relaxed meals with family and for dinner parties, so they're pretty all-purpose and work because they feel familiar. Dishes such as Spiced Sweet Potato Stew, Mushroom Risotto with Basil Cream and Spicy Lentil and Eggplant Pasta (pages 170, 184 and 193) are similar to what most people are used to eating, so your guests won't be put off just because the ingredients sound a bit alien and decide they won't like it before they even try it.

They work as well for four people as they do for twelve and can as easily be served in simple bowls on the sofa as they can on fancy plates in the dining room. They are popular among all my friends, no matter what their dietary preferences. The recipes are good and hearty

and no one realizes that they're missing meat, gluten and dairy; they finish the meal satisfied. Even if you have a total carnivore coming to dinner, these meals should go down a treat.

The other awesome thing about almost all these dishes is that they can be frozen. This means you can make one just for yourself, enjoy a serving, then stash the rest in the freezer, in portions, for a rainy day when you're too tired, stressed or tight on time to cook. I find it really helps me stay healthy if I have homemade "ready meals" in the freezer, as it means I'm never tempted to just eat raw chocolate, Gooey Black Bean Brownies (page 201) and dates for dinner! The only recipes that can't be frozen are the Creamy Carbonara and the Spicy Lentil and Eggplant Pasta (pages 190 and 193), just because pasta doesn't freeze well. But you can still make the sauces for both and freeze them, so all you have to do next time is cook a bowl of pasta, which is the easiest thing in the world.

These recipes do take a little while to cook, which is something that sets them apart from the speedier recipes in the Easy Weekday Dinners chapter. Most of them need time to allow the veggies and grains to cook and absorb all the delicious flavors. On the plus side, in general, the prep takes very little time, just ten minutes or so of chopping and throwing things together, then letting the recipe cook itself while you relax, entertain guests or get on with your to-do list! That's partly why these are so great for feeding lots of people, as it makes no difference whether you're cooking for two or twenty, you'll barely spend any more time in the kitchen;

the only change will be that you'll need more ingredients and a much bigger pan! (I use a large cast-iron pan that can go from stovetop to oven, which is perfect for this kind of cooking.) The Chickpea, Quinoa and Turmeric Curry (page 173), for example, requires almost no chopping; the only thing you have to do with a knife is cut some potatoes in half. And while I don't have any children, I hope that all my amazing readers with hungry little mouths to feed find these easy recipes especially helpful for satisfying everyone in their beautiful families without too much stress.

DINNER PARTY SUGGESTIONS

As mentioned, these recipes work well for dinner parties, so I thought it would be helpful to share some full menu ideas, so you can make your guests a feast!

Girls' Kitchen Supper

When I have girlfriends over I like to keep things really simple so I can spend time chatting with them, which is why I often choose a menu like this. It's simple enough that I don't have to stress about getting the cooking right, but it still has so much flavor that everyone really enjoys it. I like serving maple and cinnamon nuts as an appetizing snack while my guests arrive, so they can nibble on something delicious while the Warming Winter Bowls cook. I then serve brownies for dessert as they're always such a winner and can be eaten with your fingers, perfect for a chilled supper. Finally, I love ending the meal with Warming Turmeric Tonic, which makes an interesting change from tea.

Cinnamon and Maple Trail Mix (page 208)

Warming Winter Bowls (page 178)

Gooey Black Bean Brownies (page 201)

Warming Turmeric Tonic (page 239)

Skeptical Carnivores' Dinner

Feeding this group a veggie meal can be a little tricky. My tactic is to focus on big, filling meals. To start, I serve my Bright Pink Soup, as it looks beautiful and is nicely filling. My Mushroom Risotto is a wonderfully hearty recipe that satisfies every sense, so no one thinks to notice that there's no meat. This dish also conforms to preconceived ideas of what risotto should look like . . . in fact I'm sure your guests would never guess it didn't contain white rice or cheese. For the same reason, I like to serve chocolate cake as dessert. It's so fun watching skeptics enjoy the whole meal and leave thinking that perhaps being veggie may not be so terrible after all!

Bright Pink Soup (page 128)

Mushroom Risotto with Basil Cream (page 184)

Chocolate Ganache Cake (page 225)

Long Lazy Party with Barely Any Cooking

There are times—we've all been in this position—when suddenly you have way too many people to feed. This is my fail-safe menu: I promise it will work perfectly every time. You will spend hardly any time cooking and nothing can really go wrong. I serve dips with crudités, as all you really have to do is throw everything into a food processor. You can even serve ready-chopped crudités and crackers, to save time. The curry cooks itself—with the exception of chopping a few potatoes—so you can spend a few minutes prepping the crumble. I have summer and winter versions and both are equally delicious!

Smoky Eggplant Dip and Spicy Turmeric Hummus with crudités (pages 65 and 66)

Chickpea, Quinoa and Turmeric Curry (page 173)

Summer Strawberry-Banana or Winter-Spiced Pear and Apple Crumble (pages 216 and 222)

We've covered most of these shopping list ingredients in other chapters, but I quickly wanted to talk to you about the wonders of coconut milk. You'll see as you look through the recipes in this chapter that I use it a lot. It love it—it tastes delicious—but, often, the real reason I use it is to add a creamy texture. Normally the creaminess in paella or risotto, for example, comes from the rice, and a little cheese in the case of risotto; but brown rice doesn't behave in the same way as white, so we need to get the creaminess from an external source. Coconut milk does the job perfectly. I add it to my curry for the same reason; it instantly changes the texture to create something that seems much more indulgent than it is! It's worth noting that some coconut milks do contain additives, so if possible buy those that are just coconut and water. I always buy the full-fat version as I think it makes any dish more delicious, but if you prefer low-fat then all the recipes will still work.

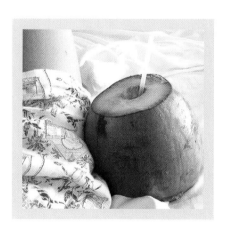

SHOPPING LIST

BLACK BEANS

CANNELLINI BEANS

CAULIFLOWER

CHIA SEEDS

CHILI FLAKES

CILANTRO

CINNAMON

COCONUT MILK

COCONUT YOGURT

CUMIN

EGGPLANT

GARLIC

MISO PASTE

MUSHROOMS

NUTRITIONAL YEAST

OLIVE OIL

PASTA (BROWN RICE)

PEAS (FROZEN)

PEPPERS

PUY LENTILS

QUINOA

RICE (SHORT-GRAIN BROWN)

SESAME OIL

SPINACH

SWEET POTATOES

TOMATOES (CANNED)

TURMERIC

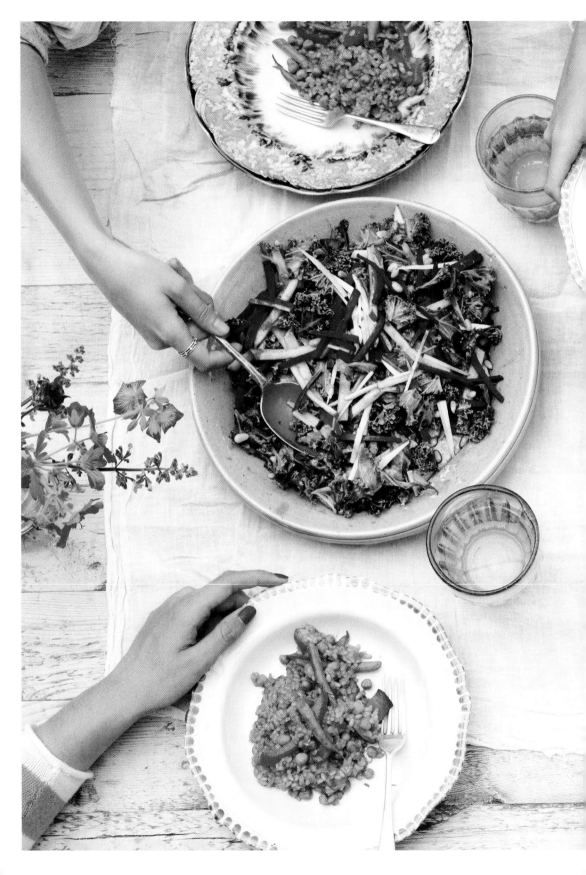

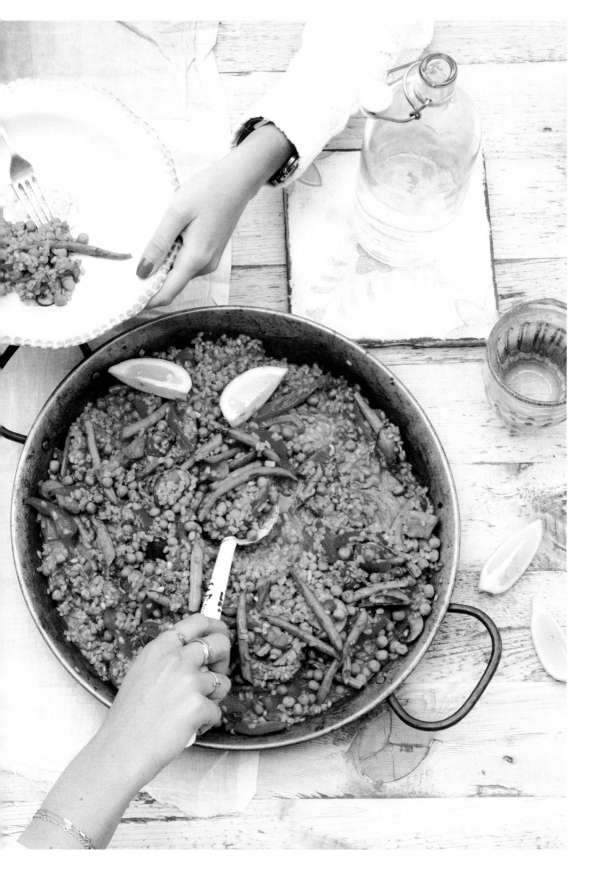

This is perfect for winter. It's an amazing dish to eat with friends from bowls on the sofa, while you cuddle under a blanket and watch a movie! The mix of sweet potatoes and black beans is nice and hearty, especially when mixed with brown rice. I love stirring coconut yogurt into this as it makes it incredibly creamy.

SPICED SWEET POTATO STEW

Serves 8

3 sweet potatoes (about 7 ounces each)
1 red bell pepper (about 4 ounces)
two 14.5-ounce cans diced tomatoes
2 garlic cloves, crushed
2 teaspoons chili powder
2 teaspoons ground cumin
2 teaspoons ground coriander
1 tablespoon miso paste
salt and pepper
one 15-ounce can black beans, drained and rinsed
7 ounces spinach
1 cup (8 ounces) coconut yogurt (optional but amazing!)

Peel the sweet potatoes, then chop them into very small (about ¾-inch) pieces. Chop the red pepper into pieces of the same size, discarding its ribs and seeds.

Place the sweet potatoes and red pepper into a large saucepan with the canned tomatoes and 2½ cups of boiling water, then bring it all to a boil.

As it boils, add the garlic, chili powder, cumin, coriander, miso paste, salt and pepper. Reduce the heat to a simmer, put the lid on the pan and allow it to cook for about 1 hour, making sure to stir it about every 5 minutes.

Now the sweet potatoes should be soft. Add the black beans to the stew with the spinach and coconut yogurt, if using, and stir well until the spinach has wilted totally. (Or serve the coconut yogurt on top, instead, as we did for the photograph.)

Tweak It

If you don't have coconut yogurt and you're OK eating dairy, use Greek yogurt instead; make sure it's full-fat though as it's much creamier and thicker, which makes this more delicious.

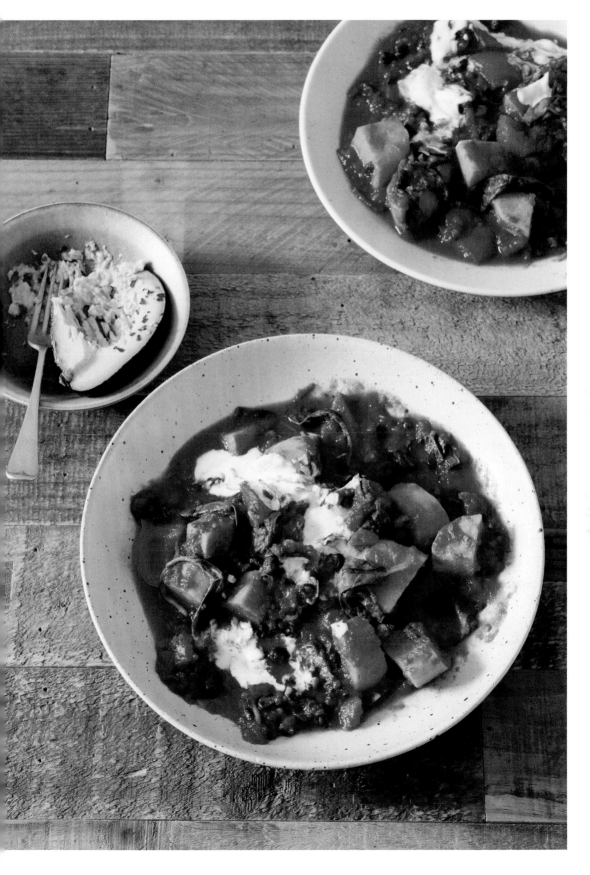

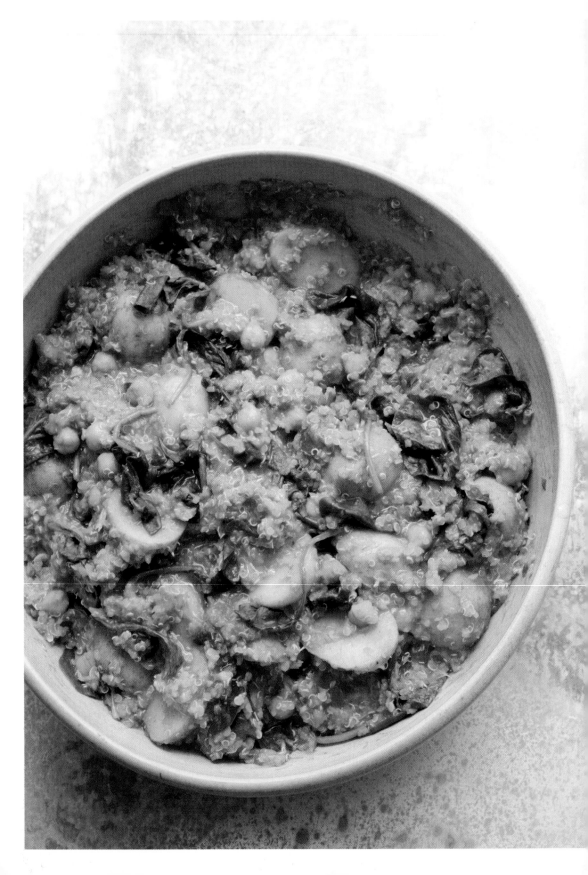

The first recipe I created for this book, this is still one of my favorites! I've made it for almost everyone I know and get constant requests from friends for it when they come over, it's so popular. The thing that makes it so delicious is that the quinoa is cooked in the coconut curry blend, so it soaks in all the incredible flavors. This means that each bite is bursting with the tastes of turmeric, coriander, ginger, garlic and chili. The spinach adds a beautiful color, its vibrant green creating a great contrast to the yellowy-orange curry.

CHICKPEA, QUINOA AND TURMERIC CURRY

Serves 6

1 pound new potatoes, halved
3 garlic cloves, crushed
1 tablespoon ground turmeric
1 teaspoon ground coriander
1 teaspoon chili flakes or powder
1 teaspoon ground ginger
one 14-ounce can coconut milk
1 tablespoon tomato paste
one 14.5-ounce can diced
  tomatoes
salt and pepper
1 cup quinoa
one 14-ounce can chickpeas,
  drained and rinsed
5 ounces spinach

Place the potatoes in a pan of cold water and bring to a boil, then let them cook for about 25 minutes, until you can easily stick a knife through them. Drain them well.

Place the potatoes in a large pan and add the garlic, turmeric, coriander, chili, ginger, coconut milk, tomato paste and chopped tomatoes. Bring to a boil, season with salt and pepper, then add the quinoa and 1⅔ cups just-boiled water.

Reduce the heat to a simmer, place the lid on and allow to cook. Over the next 30 minutes, stir every 5 minutes or so to make sure nothing sticks to the bottom. (This is quite a long cooking time, but this is how long quinoa takes to cook with all these ingredients, rather than just in water.) Halfway through cooking, add the chickpeas. When there are just 5 minutes left, add the spinach and stir it in until it wilts. Once the quinoa has cooked and is fluffy, not crunchy, it's ready.

Kitchen Know-How

Be so careful with turmeric, it stains everything. Wear an apron while making this, try not to leave turmeric-coated spoons on white surfaces and don't spill it over anything!

Tweak It

If you like a bit of heat, add a sliced red chili to the cooking curry at the same time as the other spices.

This may be my favorite recipe for feeding a crowd; I absolutely adore it. Each bite is bursting with so much flavor and everyone I've served this to loves it, including a Spanish man, which says a lot! I was inspired to make this by a dish I tried in Colombia that was made from brown rice, spices and coconut milk; I loved it so much that I've been experimenting with the combination ever since and this is my best version!

VEGGIE PAELLA

Serves 4

2 red bell peppers, sliced
7 ounces cremini mushrooms, chopped
1½ cups frozen peas
7 ounces green beans, ends trimmed
2 teaspoons cayenne pepper
4 teaspoons paprika
juice of 3 lemons, plus more lemons to serve
olive oil
4 garlic cloves, crushed
salt
about 24 cherry tomatoes
1 teaspoon saffron threads
2⅔ cups short-grain brown rice
one 14-ounce can coconut milk
small bunch of cilantro (about ½ ounce), finely chopped

Add the red peppers and mushrooms to a large saucepan with the peas, green beans, cayenne, paprika, the juice of 1 lemon, a generous amount of olive oil, the garlic and salt. Cook for about 5 minutes, until the veggies are starting to soften.

Meanwhile, chop the tomatoes into quarters.

Add the tomatoes and saffron to the pan, then, a couple of minutes later, stir in the rice and coconut milk, adding 3 cups of water.

Place the lid on the pan and bring the paella to a boil, then reduce the heat to a simmer. Let it cook for 1 hour. Try not to stir it too much during this time, just every 20 minutes or so to ensure the rice isn't sticking to the bottom of the pan.

After 1 hour the rice should feel cooked but still a little al dente. Stir in the juice of the remaining 2 lemons.

Place the paella in bowls, with lemon wedges on the side, sprinkling the chopped cilantro on top.

Tweak It

If you want to make this heartier, stir in some boiled potatoes halfway through. Or, if you're a fish eater, add some fish fillets or shrimp to it, too, 5–10 minutes before the end of cooking.

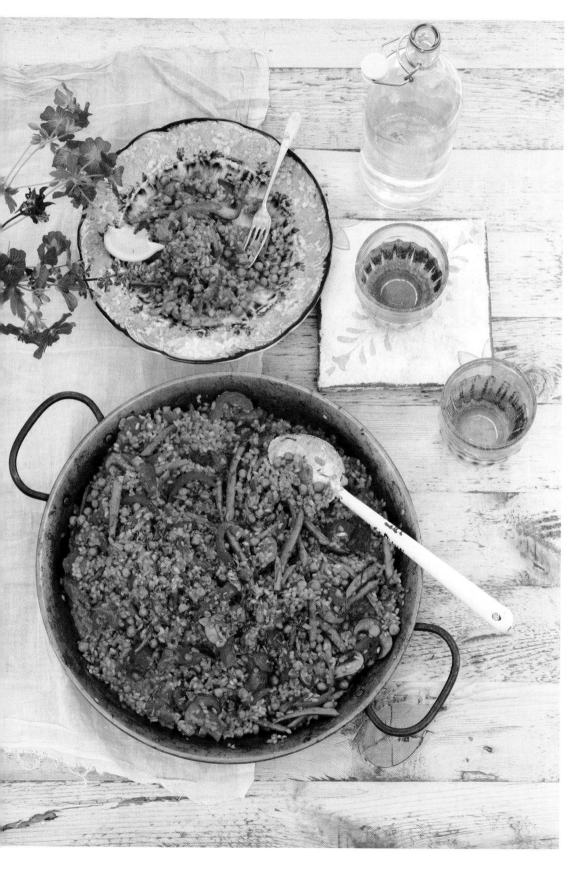

This is so nourishing and delicious. It's the perfect comfort food as it's so satisfying and packed with an amazing mix of flavors. Each bite is full of wilted spinach, toasted pine nuts and tender chunks of sweet potato, which all melt into the coconut-infused rice. I love this served with my Simple Cucumber and Tomato Salad or Green Beans and Salsa (pages 104 and 108); each complements the risotto perfectly!

CREAMY SWEET POTATO RISOTTO

Serves 6

For the rice

2⅔ cups short-grain brown rice
one 14-ounce can coconut milk
2 tablespoons apple cider vinegar
salt

For the sauce

4 sweet potatoes (9 ounces each)
4 tablespoons olive oil, plus more
    to serve (optional)
salt and pepper
1 teaspoon ground cinnamon
¾ cup pine nuts
1 tablespoon apple cider vinegar
2 tablespoons tahini
1 tablespoon sesame oil
3 tablespoons nutritional yeast
1 tablespoon ground cumin
juice of 1 lemon
3 garlic cloves, roughly chopped
handful of cilantro, finely
    chopped
7 ounces spinach

Preheat the oven to 350°F (convection 325°F).

Put the rice into a large saucepan with 3 cups of water. Pour in the coconut milk and vinegar and add salt. Bring it to a boil and, once it has boiled for a minute or so, reduce the heat to a simmer. Cover and cook for about 45 minutes, until the rice has cooked and all the liquid has been absorbed.

Meanwhile, chop 3 of the sweet potatoes into bite-size pieces, place them on a baking sheet with a tablespoon of the olive oil, salt, pepper and the cinnamon. Put the baking sheet in the oven and cook for 30 minutes. Just before the end of cooking, add the pine nuts and let them cook for a couple of minutes until they're golden brown.

At the same time, peel the remaining sweet potato, cut it into small bite-size pieces and place in a steamer for 15 minutes, until really soft.

Once the steamed sweet potato is cooked, add it to a blender with the 3 tablespoons of olive oil, a scant ½ cup of water, the vinegar, tahini, sesame oil, nutritional yeast, cumin, lemon juice, garlic, salt and pepper. Blend until a smooth mixture forms.

Once the rice has finished cooking, stir in the blended mixture along with the roasted sweet potato chunks, pine nuts, cilantro and spinach. Let this cook together until the spinach has wilted, then serve. I like drizzling a little olive oil over each serving.

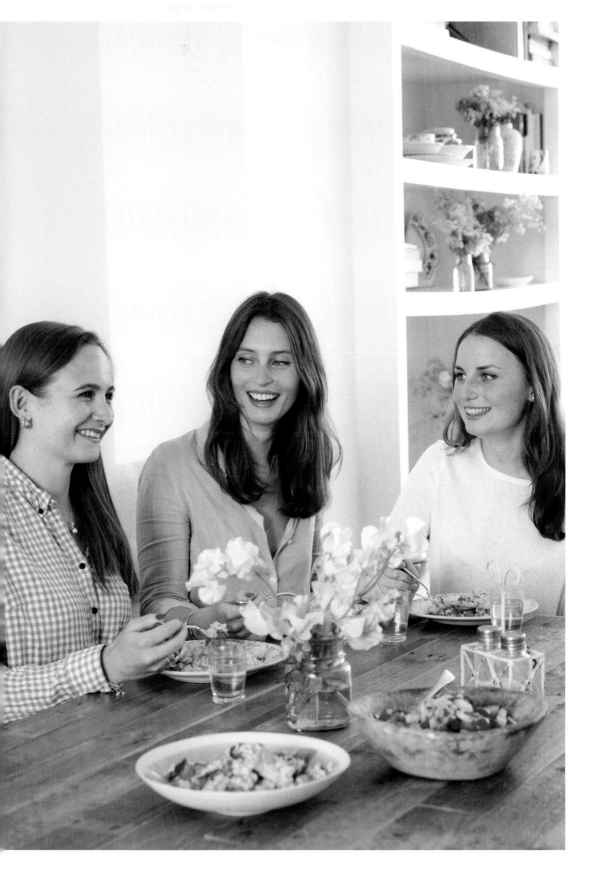

When the weather is cold, I find myself craving this beautiful combination of flavors all the time. I just love how the cinnamon, ginger, tamari and lime blend together to infuse all the veggies and legumes. The mix of lentils, cannellini beans and carrots makes a wonderfully filling, hearty meal—especially when served with brown rice—that will warm you up from the inside out.

WARMING WINTER BOWLS

Serves 8

5 carrots
two 14.5-ounce cans
   diced tomatoes
generous ½ cup Puy lentils
5 tablespoons tomato paste
I tablespoon plus 2 teaspoons
   tamari
I tablespoon ground cinnamon
I tablespoon ground ginger
3 garlic cloves, crushed
salt and pepper
3 zucchini
two 15-ounce cans cannellini
   beans, drained and rinsed
juice of I lime

Start by peeling the carrots, then slicing them into thin rounds. If they are quite fat, cut the rounds in half. Place them into a large saucepan.

Add the diced tomatoes, lentils, tomato paste, tamari, cinnamon, ginger, garlic, salt and pepper to the saucepan, then pour in 2½ cups of boiling water and mix everything together. Bring to a boil, then reduce the heat to a simmer, place the lid on the pan and let it simmer for 30 minutes.

Slice the zucchini into half-moons, then stir them into the saucepan along with the cannellini beans and lime juice and let everything simmer for another 30–40 minutes, until the carrots and zucchini are nice and soft.

Tweak It

If you feel like an extra hit of greens, try stirring a bag of spinach into the saucepan just before it finishes cooking.

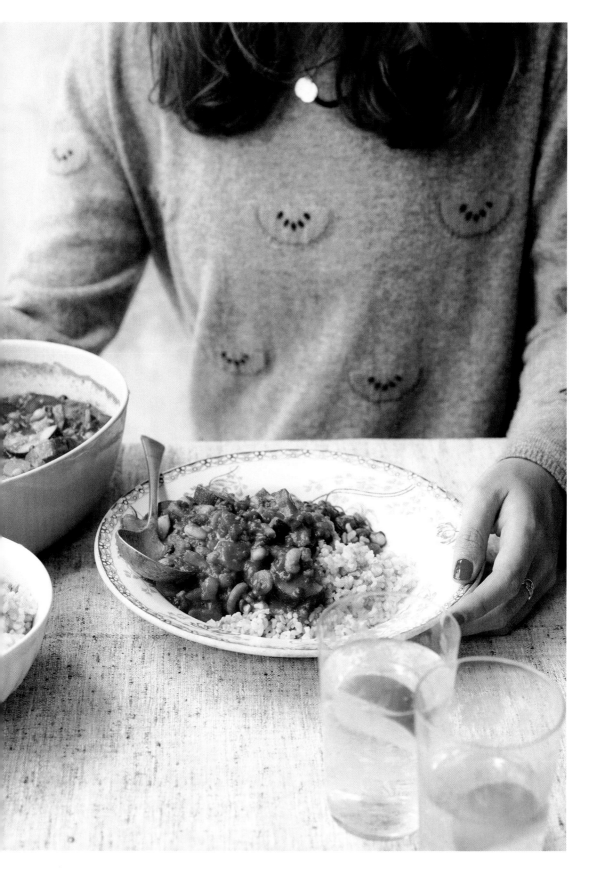

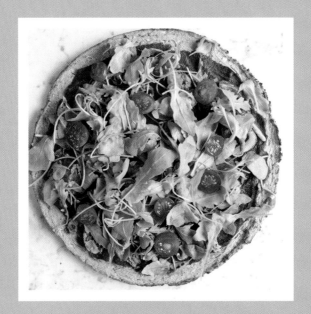

ARUGULA LEAVES ADD
FRESH GREEN GOODNESS

If you're a pizza lover, this recipe is going to make you so happy! I know the idea of using cauliflower as a pizza base may sound strange, but this is the best healthy crust I've come across; it really is amazing. Even the skeptics have loved it!

CAULIFLOWER PIZZA

Makes 2 large pizza crusts / Serves 4–6

¼ cup chia seeds
2 heads of cauliflower (about 2¼ pounds total), roughly chopped
scant 1 cup Apple Purée (page 40)
1¾ cups plus 2 tablespoons brown rice flour or buckwheat flour
juice of 2 lemons
2 tablespoons tamari
salt
4 teaspoons dried oregano
4 teaspoons dried basil

For the toppings, I like:

tomato paste
sliced tomatoes
canned corn
sliced mushrooms
fresh basil leaves
handful of arugula
salt and pepper
olive oil

Place the chia seeds in a bowl with a scant 1¼ cups of water. Leave for 10–15 minutes, until the chia has formed a gel.

Preheat the oven to 400°F (convection 350°F).

Place the cauliflower in a food processor and blend it until a flour-like substance forms; this should take about a minute (you may need to do this in 2 batches). Place in a nut milk bag (page 53) and knead out excess water: it may take a few minutes but it's a really important step, so please don't skip it!

Add the cauliflower to a mixing bowl with the chia and apple purée and stir until blended. Mix in the flour, lemon juice, tamari, salt and dried herbs. Slowly pour in ½ cup plus 2 tablespoons of ice-cold water, using your hands to mix it to a sticky dough. Divide the dough into 2 pieces.

Line 2 baking sheets with parchment paper and spread each piece of dough out over it, to form a pizza base. Bake the crusts for 20–30 minutes.

Once they are firm and slightly crispy, add the tomato paste and your toppings (except any fresh herbs such as basil or arugula), then cook for another 5–10 minutes. Sprinkle with salt and pepper, any fresh herbs and a drizzle of olive oil, then slice and serve!

Kitchen Know-How

I know it sounds strange to tell you to take the water out of the cauliflower and then add more water to the mixture, but—trust me—it's vital for the recipe to work, as it means you get exactly the right amount of liquid needed for the crust to bake properly.

My favorite post-workout dinner, these really take just ten minutes to throw together and they're so satisfying! If you have lots of hungry friends coming over, then these are a lovely, easy meal that will keep everyone happy. I love serving them on a bed of sautéed spinach, or with salad, with a big bowl of Sweet Potato Wedges (page 187) on the side.

BLACK BEAN BURGERS

Makes 8

two 15-ounce cans black beans,
   drained and rinsed
generous 1 cup chickpea flour
3 tablespoons tomato paste
2 tablespoons Apple Purée
   (page 40)
1 teaspoon chili powder
2 teaspoons tamari
2 teaspoons apple cider vinegar
juice of ½ lime
salt and pepper
coconut oil, to shallow-fry

Put the beans in a large mixing bowl. Mash them with a fork until they're pretty mushy, but not totally smooth; there should still be some whole beans in the mixture.

Stir in all the remaining ingredients, except the coconut oil.

Heat a saucepan with a little coconut oil, then place 1 heaping tablespoon of the mixture into the center of the pan. Shape it into a round and then spread it out a little so it's about ¾ inch thick. Repeat to form 4 burgers in the pan. Let the burgers cook for about 1 minute on each side, flipping them so that they cook evenly.

Then do the same thing with the remaining burger mixture, keeping the cooked burgers warm while you cook the rest.

Kitchen Know-How

I know the apple purée might sound like a weird ingredient, but please don't leave it out; it really helps the burgers stick together and it adds a delicious flavor!

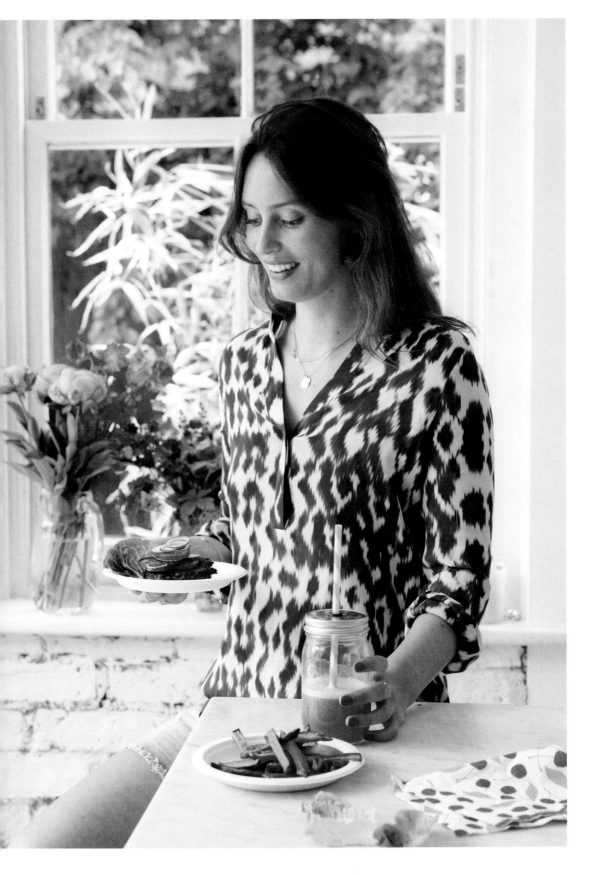

Definitely one of my most used recipes in the book. Before I became a healthy eater, risotto was my go-to comfort food and I missed it so much when I changed my diet. It's taken me a while to perfect a healthy risotto, but this is it. I love stirring in the basil cream to make it extra-indulgent and comforting, plus it adds a beautiful flavor to each bite. This is great for larger numbers, because you don't need to stir it constantly, as you do with many risottos.

MUSHROOM RISOTTO WITH BASIL CREAM

Serves 6

For the risotto

6 garlic cloves, crushed
4 teaspoons dried thyme
4 teaspoons dried oregano
2 teaspoons ground cumin
6 tablespoons olive oil
1 pound cremini mushrooms, sliced
two 14-ounce cans coconut milk
2⅔ cups short-grain brown rice
juice of 2 limes
salt and pepper
juice of 2 lemons
¾ cup frozen peas

For the basil cream

small bunch of fresh basil (about 1 cup)
2 garlic cloves, peeled
generous ½ cup pine nuts
5 tablespoons olive oil
juice of 1 lemon

Place the crushed garlic, thyme, oregano, cumin and olive oil in a large saucepan. Heat this gently for a minute or so, then stir in the mushrooms. Cook for another 2–3 minutes, so they are coated in the herbs, spices and garlic.

Mix 3 cups of boiling water into the mushrooms with 1 can of coconut milk, the rice, lime juice, salt and pepper. Place the lid on the pan, bring it to a boil and, once it has boiled for a minute or so, reduce the heat to a simmer. Leave to simmer for 45 minutes, stirring it once or twice during this time.

When the rice is almost cooked, stir in the remaining can of coconut milk, the lemon juice and peas. Cook for another 15 minutes or so, until the rice tastes perfect.

Meanwhile, make the basil cream. Simply pull the basil leaves from their stems. Place all the ingredients into a food processor, pour in a scant 2 tablespoons of water and a little salt and blend until smooth.

Once the risotto has finished cooking, place it into bowls and stir a spoonful of the basil cream into each serving.

Tweak It

If you don't have the ingredients for the basil cream, don't worry, the dish is still so delicious without it! You can also add extra color, texture and green goodness by stirring in a bag of spinach at the end.

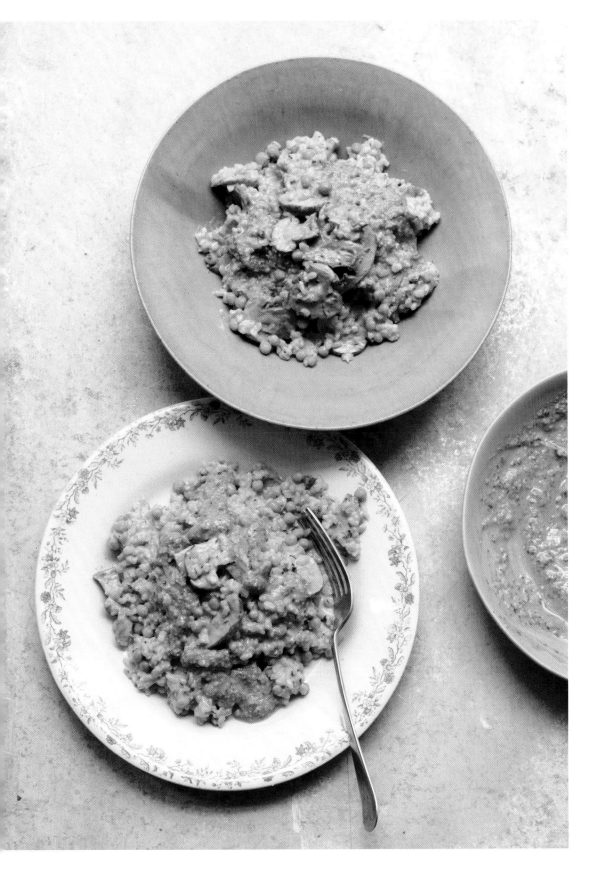

A wonderful all-rounder dish. It works so well as a main course served over brown rice or pasta, but it's equally great as a side dish with just about anything. I love making big batches of this on a Sunday night and keeping portions of it in the freezer, as it's such an easy addition to any weeknight meal, plus it's so simple to make in the first place.

EASY RATATOUILLE

Serves 4

4 large tomatoes

2 eggplants

2 zucchini

2 red bell peppers

4 garlic cloves

¼ cup olive oil

I tablespoon herbes de Provence

I tablespoon dried thyme

3 tablespoons tomato paste

I teaspoon honey

juice of I lime

2 teaspoons tamari

I teaspoon chili powder

2 teaspoons paprika

Score a line across the bottom of the tomatoes, then place them in a saucepan of boiling water and let them heat for about 30 seconds. Drain the water and rinse the tomatoes with cold water before peeling the skins off. Chop them into small pieces, discarding the skins and seedy centers.

Chop all the other veggies into large bite-size chunks.

Crush the garlic into a saucepan with the olive oil and herbs and let them cook for a couple of minutes so that they're bubbling. Then add all the veggies.

Place the lid on the pan and let it simmer over medium heat for 30 minutes, at which point all the veggies should be nice and soft.

Finally stir in the tomato paste, honey, lime juice, tamari, chili powder and paprika. Let everything cook together for a minute or so, then serve.

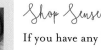

Shop Sense

If you have any leftover veggies in the fridge, you can add those to the mix, too. I add grated carrot, sautéed broccoli, any green leafy veg and so on to the pot and it's always great!

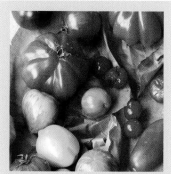

Adapted from one of my favorite blog recipes and it was good before . . . but now it's even better! I normally serve my stews and curries with brown rice, but one day I ran out of rice and tried serving this with sweet potato wedges instead. It was such a revelation; they add so much flavor and a wonderful tender texture to each bite.

KALE AND CANNELLINI STEW WITH SWEET POTATO WEDGES

Serves 4

4 medium or 3 large
   sweet potatoes
olive oil
salt and pepper
7 ounces kale
3 garlic cloves, finely sliced
one 9.9-ounce jar oil-packed
   sun-dried tomatoes, drained
   and roughly chopped
two 14.5-ounce cans
   diced tomatoes
one 15-ounce can cannellini
   beans, drained and rinsed
2 tablespoons tomato paste
1 tablespoon tahini
1 tablespoon apple cider vinegar
1 teaspoon chili flakes

Preheat the oven to 350°F (convection 325°F).

Chop the sweet potatoes into wedges and place them on a baking sheet with a little olive oil and a sprinkling of salt. Let them cook for about 1 hour, until they're tender, turning halfway though.

Once the sweet potatoes have cooked for about 40 minutes, start making the rest of the stew: tear the leaves of the kale from the stems and discard the stems.

Heat a little more olive oil in a large saucepan and lightly fry the garlic for 30 seconds, then add the kale leaves. Sauté, turning often, for a couple of minutes.

Add the drained, chopped sun-dried tomatoes with all the other ingredients. Cook for about 10 minutes, until the kale is nice and soft, then season with salt and pepper.

Serve by pouring the stew over the sweet potato wedges.

Tweak It

If you don't have sweet potatoes—or want to add a different flavor under the stew—try using parsnips and potatoes either instead of, or as well as, the sweet potatoes.

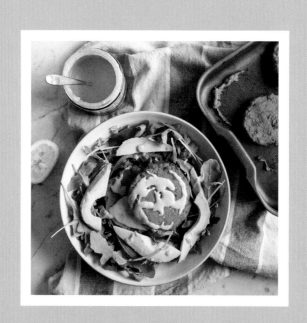

GLOWING GLOBES
OF GORGEOUSNESS

One of my oldest and most-loved recipes. I first made these shortly after I changed my diet and I'm still making them now, which says a lot about how great this recipe is! I love serving them on a big bed of arugula and avocado with a generous drizzling of tahini, olive oil and lots of lime juice; it's a marvelous dinner. If you're making these for a roomful of guests, try accompanying them with my Sesame Marinated Kale or Perfect Pesto Veggies (pages 75 and 84).

MY FAVORITE SWEET POTATO CAKES

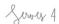

Serves 4

4 sweet potatoes
2 tablespoons quinoa flour, buckwheat flour or brown rice flour, plus more to dust
2 tablespoons tomato paste
2 garlic cloves, crushed
handful of cilantro, finely chopped
I teaspoon ground cumin
I teaspoon chili flakes
I heaping tablespoon tahini
juice of I lime, plus lime wedges to serve
salt and pepper
olive oil, for the baking sheet

Peel the sweet potatoes and cut them into bite-size chunks. Place these in a steamer and steam until they are very soft; this should take about 15 minutes.

Preheat the oven to 425°F (convection 400°F).

Place the steamed potatoes in a bowl and mash them with a fork until they are nearly smooth. Stir in the flour, tomato paste, garlic, cilantro, cumin, chili flakes, tahini, lime juice, salt and pepper. Mix everything together. It's a good idea to chill the mixture at this point to firm it up, but don't worry if you haven't got the time as it will still work fine.

Mold the mixture into 4 even cakes.

Dust the top of each cake with flour (this is what makes the outsides crispy) and place the cakes on an oiled baking sheet.

Bake for about 20 minutes, until the tops start to turn a golden brown and the cakes are no longer sticky. Serve with lime wedges.

Kitchen Know-How

If you're trying to eat less fish, but you're a fish cake lover, this recipe is for you! I first made them as I was missing salmon fish cakes and they filled that void perfectly . . . in fact I actually thought they were way more delicious.

I've been working on this recipe for so long! Growing up, I was obsessed with cheesy pasta and I missed it so much when I changed my diet, so I've spent the last two years trying to replicate the same creamy, comforting dish but with a nourishing element. This is the final result, which I adore. I make this a lot for friends and it's always a big hit!

CREAMY CARBONARA

Serves 4

For the sauce

5 ounces cashews
⅓ butternut squash (about 7 ounces)
2 teaspoons nutritional yeast
I tablespoon tamari
½ teaspoon cayenne pepper
juice of I lemon
salt and lots of pepper

For the pasta

brown rice pasta (about 3.5 ounces per person, or according to appetite!)
¾ cup frozen peas
2 garlic cloves, crushed
7 ounces mushrooms, finely sliced
olive oil
7 ounces spinach

Soak the cashews in a bowl of water for 3–4 hours.

Peel and chop the squash, place it in a steamer and steam it for 15 minutes, until really soft.

Discard the water that the cashews have been soaking in, then tip them into a blender with the steamed squash and all the remaining sauce ingredients. Pour in a generous ¾ cup of water and blitz everything together.

Put the pasta in a pan of boiling water and cook according to the package instructions. Add the peas 2 minutes before the end of cooking time.

While they cook, sauté the garlic and mushrooms in a little olive oil, adding the spinach toward the end so that it wilts.

Once the peas and pasta are cooked, drain them, then mix them with the sauce, mushrooms and spinach to serve.

Make It Better

If you want to make this lighter, try using Zucchini Noodles (page 83) instead of conventional pasta.

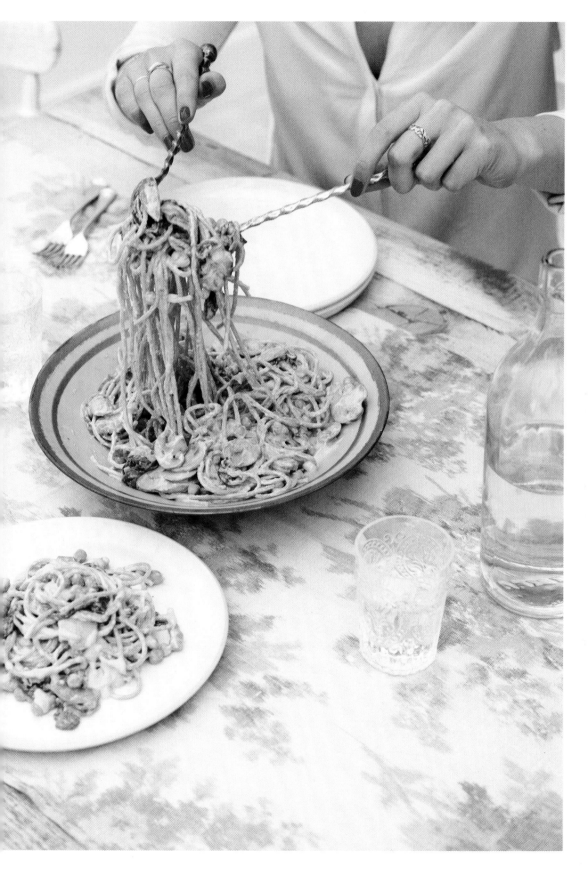

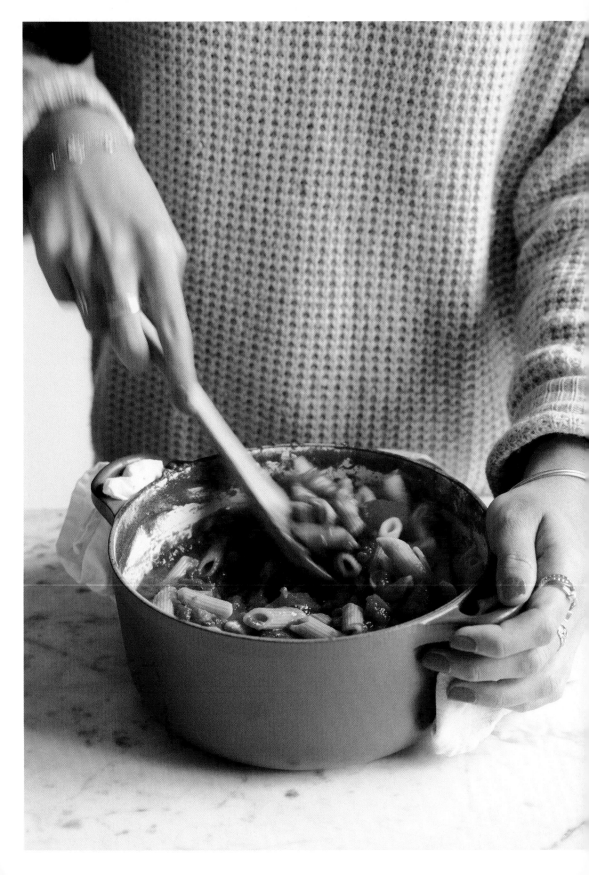

When I'm feeling lazy and have lots of people to feed, I head straight for this pasta recipe. It's so warming and comforting and everyone always loves it as it feels very familiar, not healthy and scary! It's the easiest recipe, too: all you have to do is chop up some eggplants and red pepper and throw them in a pan to simmer with lentils, canned tomatoes and spices (and then boil some pasta).

SPICY LENTIL AND EGGPLANT PASTA

Serves 6

2 eggplants
1 red bell pepper
two 14.5-ounce cans
    diced tomatoes
1 tablespoon tomato paste
1 teaspoon chili flakes
2 teaspoons paprika
1 tablespoon cumin seeds
1 tablespoon tamari
2 garlic cloves, finely chopped
generous ½ cup Puy lentils
2 teaspoons tahini
1 pound brown rice pasta

Slice the eggplants and red pepper into small bite-size pieces and place them in a large saucepan with all the remaining ingredients, except the tahini and pasta. Pour in 1½ cups of boiling water.

Place over medium heat, then return to a boil. Reduce the heat to a simmer, put on a lid and cook for about 1 hour. Stir in the tahini.

About 10 minutes before the lentils are ready, cook the pasta according to the package instructions. Drain, then stir it into the eggplant sauce.

Tweak It

If you want to switch this up, or don't like eggplant, try replacing them with another veggie. I find that zucchini works really well.

GOOEY BLACK BEAN BROWNIES

GINGERBREAD COOKIES

ENERGY BITES, TWO WAYS

CACAO, OAT AND RAISIN COOKIES

QUINOA AND CACAO CRISPY TREATS

TRAIL MIX, TWO WAYS

CINNAMON-COCONUT POPCORN

SIMPLE SWEETS

COCONUT AND RASPBERRY MOUSSE

SUMMER STRAWBERRY-BANANA CRUMBLE

CHOCOLATE AND HAZELNUT TARTS

WINTER-SPICED PEAR AND APPLE CRUMBLE

CHOCOLATE GANACHE CAKE

PECAN PIE

DOUBLE-CHOCOLATE CHEESECAKE BROWNIES

CHOCOLATE CARAMEL SLICES

SPICED FRUIT BOWLS

BAOBAB TRUFFLES

HOT CHOCOLATE

WARM BEET AND APPLE JUICE

WARMING TURMERIC TONIC

SPICY HONEY LEMON TEA

FRESH MINT TEA

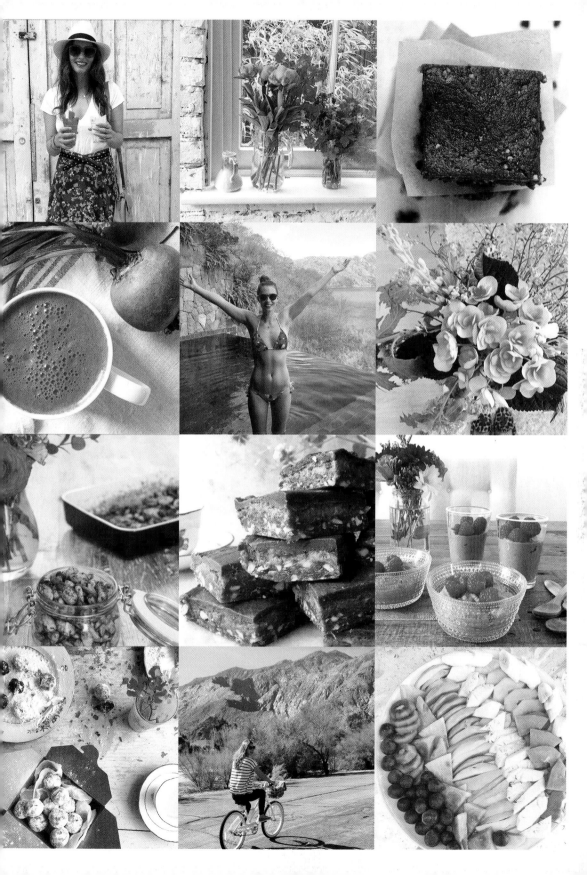

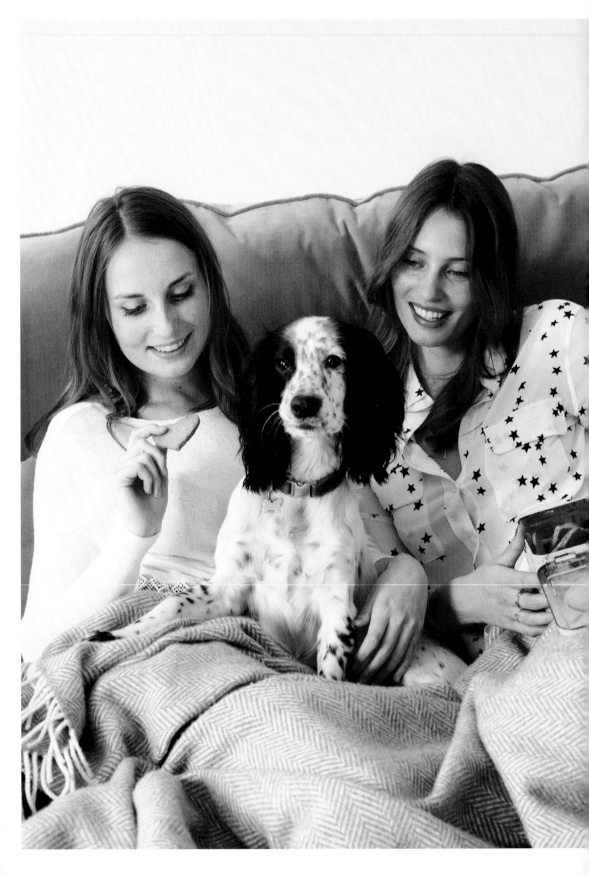

SIMPLE SWEETS

As many of my blog readers will know, I have a big sweet tooth, I always have had and I'm pretty sure I always will! However, my sweet tooth has changed quite dramatically since I transformed my diet. I still want something sweet most days, but the desire now comes in a different form. Over time my palate has changed. I no longer get excited about refined sugar, but instead crave Gooey Black Bean Brownies, Cinnamon and Honey Energy Bites and Warm Beet and Apple Juice (pages 201, 204 and 236), which is a big change from my days of wanting slabs of cheap chocolate and candy.

When you're changing your diet and shifting toward a more natural way of eating, it's important to be a bit organized and have sweet snacks on hand, so you reach for those rather than the candy jar! That's where these recipes come in: they're easy to make and most of them last for a while, so you can stock your kitchen with treats to keep you prepared at all times.

I've focused on three different types of sweets in this chapter: those to enjoy on-the-go, desserts to serve to friends and soothing drinks to satisfy a subtle sweet tooth. The on-the-go section is about snacks that you can easily carry around with you, such as Cacao, Oat and Raisin Cookies and Quinoa and Cacao Crispy Treats (pages 205 and 206). These are awesome afternoon pick-me-ups that work to fight off the four o'clock slump as they boost your energy levels, keep your mood stable and help stave off the cravings for snacks high in refined sugar. This is because they're full of plant protein, healthy fats and lots of fiber.

Plant protein is so important for keeping you energized, as every cell needs it to function, plus it's vital to maintain your biological processes, such as digestion. In addition to these roles, protein signals to your brain that you're full, so it's great to include it in your snacks. Fiber also boosts protein's ability to energize you, as the more fiber something contains, the slower it is released into your blood stream; therefore you stay satisfied for longer and your blood sugar levels stay on an even keel so you won't get any aggressive hunger pangs! I'd really recommend keeping some of these on-the-go snacks in your desk at work, taking them to school or keeping them in your bag while you run around, as they'll truly help to keep your energy levels boosted all day.

Of course, you can absolutely serve on-the-go sweets to friends, too. I've found they are really popular, especially the brownies, which are a favorite of mine for cozy dinners in with my girlfriends. However, most of the sweets that I love to share look more like traditional desserts, as I think it's nice to serve them in a beautiful dish or plate so everyone can help themselves to a slice or a portion. I love things such as Coconut and Raspberry Mousse, Chocolate and Hazelnut Tarts and Pecan Pie (pages 215, 219 and 226). These dishes aren't super-portable, though, so I'd really stick to the snacks section if you're looking for sweet treats that are easy to pack up and take with you for the day, and save the other recipes for dessert on occasions when you want to impress your friends at a lunch or dinner party.

I've also included warming drinks here, as I love finishing dinner with something sweet, but I don't always want a dessert. They are all great immune boosters if you're feeling a little cold, sleepy or slightly under the weather: they'll warm your whole body up from the inside out, leaving you feeling rejuvenated.

I'll make mugs of creamy Hot Chocolate, Warm Beet and Apple Juice or Warming Turmeric Tonic to keep my sweet tooth in check (pages 235, 236 and 239) and find they do wonders for my happiness levels. They're also a gentle way to finish a meal and often help with digestion, especially the Spicy Honey Lemon Tea (page 240). If you're feeling too full, a mug of this should help!

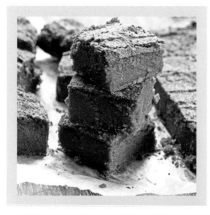

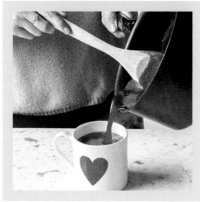

MY FAVORITE SWEET INGREDIENTS

I've told you about oats, apples and chia seeds in the Breakfast chapter, so I'll quickly run through why I keep my pantry stocked with some of the other ingredients on my sweet shopping list.

Flours—brown rice and buckwheat are my go-to flours; both gluten-free and full of fiber, vitamins and minerals. I find they work in every recipe. They also last for ages, so you can keep your pantry stocked. As I've tried to keep many of these recipes nut-free, you'll find that they are used in almost everything.

Black beans—I use these in my brownies, which are a staple in my house. I normally have a batch floating around the kitchen, as they're so easy to make and a great thing to feed to friends when they stop by. Black beans support your digestive system, while also giving a great protein and fiber boost, so they're amazing to eat if you're looking to increase energy levels.

Condiments—coconut oil and apple purée are essentials for my sweet recipes and are used time and time again, from the Quinoa and Cacao Crispy Treats to the Spiced Fruit Bowls and the Baobab Truffles (pages 206, 231 and 232). Both help ingredients to bind together, while adding subtle sweetness. Coconut oil is easy to find but apple purée isn't as widely available, so I make it myself (page 40).

Sweeteners—my favorites are raw honey, date syrup and maple syrup. All three are natural and won't spike your blood sugar in the same way that white sugar does, plus they all have nutritious properties. Honey is wonderfully anti-inflammatory, date syrup is full of fiber, while maple syrup contains an array of vitamins and minerals including zinc and magnesium. Maple syrup is the runniest, so is normally easiest to use in baking, whereas both date syrup and raw honey are really sticky . . . this can be helpful in getting mixes to stick together, which is why I use them in Cacao, Oat and Raisin Cookies and Winter-Spiced Pear and Apple Crumble topping (pages 205 and 222). It's worth noting that these are all more expensive than refined sugar and sadly there's not really a way to make them cheaper. I normally only bake once a week, though, and don't spend money on chocolate bars, so I find the cost evens out over the week.

Dried fruits—especially raisins and medjool dates. I use both quite often to sweeten food. Raisins also add a juicy bite to whatever you're eating, which I love, especially in Gooey Black Bean Brownies and Cacao, Oat and Raisin Cookies (pages 201 and 205). As with the natural sweeteners, dried fruit can be quite pricey, so, if possible, try to buy it in bulk.

Dry goods—raw cacao powder, almonds, pecans and cashews. Raw cacao is one of my all-time favorite ingredients and you will need it for all the chocolatey recipes in this chapter. It is the unprocessed version of cocoa, so it has much more goodness in it and also a much stronger flavor so you need to use less of it than regular cocoa powder. So, although it's more expensive to buy, it actually works out cheaper as it goes so much further. Almonds, pecans and cashews are important, too, as they're my favorite nuts to cook with, so you'll find they pop up quite often.

SHOPPING LIST

ALMOND BUTTER

ALMONDS

APPLES

BAOBAB POWDER

BERRIES

BLACK BEANS

CACAO NIBS

CACAO POWDER (RAW)

CASHEWS

CAYENNE PEPPER

COCONUT CREAM

COCONUT OIL

COCONUT SUGAR

DATE SYRUP

DATES (MEDJOOL)

FLOUR (BROWN RICE AND BUCKWHEAT)

GINGER (FRESH)

HONEY

MAPLE SYRUP

OATS

PECANS

POPCORN

QUINOA (POPPED OR PUFFED)

RAISINS

TURMERIC

VANILLA PODS AND POWDER

SWEET SNACKS

To take on-the-go or keep in your desk drawer—
portable comfort on busy days

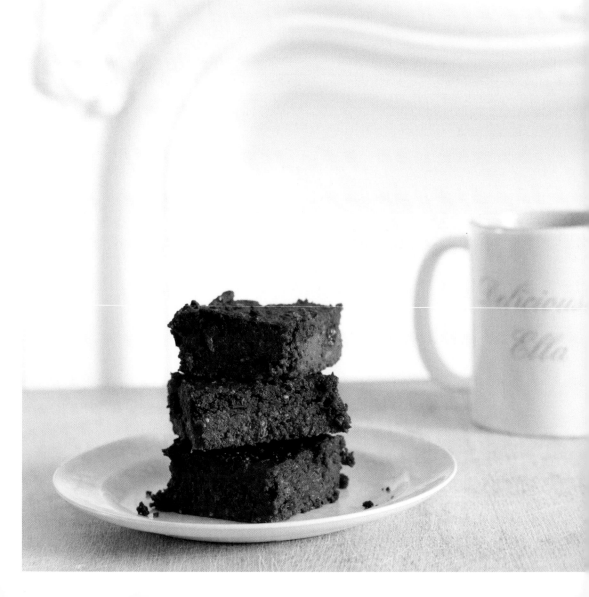

I've now created four types of brownies: sweet potato brownies, raw brownies, glazed beet chili brownies and—drum roll—these black bean brownies. The same friends have tried all versions and they loved these the best, so I hope you do, too! They're gooier than the others and the raisins give each bite a juicy plumpness. I know that beans might sound like a weird ingredient, but that's what makes the texture so great. (Don't worry, you can't taste them!) There's a fifth brownie recipe in this chapter, too, but I won't spoil it for you . . . read on to find it!

GOOEY BLACK BEAN BROWNIES

Makes 12

2 tablespoons chia seeds
one 15-ounce can black beans, drained and rinsed
2 cups almond-meal
generous ¾ cup Apple Purée (page 40)
generous ¾ cup plant-based milk (I use almond milk here)
2 tablespoons coconut oil
2 tablespoons honey
½ cup maple syrup
7–8 tablespoons raw cacao powder (use more depending on how chocolaty you like it)
pinch of salt
½ cup plus 2 tablespoons raisins

Soak the chia seeds in a generous ½ cup of water for about 30 minutes.

Preheat the oven to 350°F (convection 325°F).

Place all the ingredients—except the raisins—into a food processor and blend until smooth. Stir in the raisins until evenly mixed in.

Line a baking dish (mine was 12 x 8 x 2 inches) with parchment paper, then pour the brownie batter in and spread it out.

Bake for about 40 minutes, or until a knife comes out almost clean. Let the brownies cool for about 45 minutes in the baking dish; this is really important as they continue setting during this time. Cut into 12 brownies.

Store in an airtight container for up to 5 days.

Kitchen Know-How

It's really important that you leave these to cool as that's when they set; they're not totally solid when they come out the oven, so please have patience!

Such a great snack: nicely balanced but not too sweet and with a crunchy texture that feels so satisfying. They're really portable, too, so you can keep a few in your desk drawer to be prepared for any craving! If you want something extra-sumptuous, try spreading some Cashew and Vanilla Butter (page 39) over them, it's divine!

GINGERBREAD COOKIES

Makes 16

3.5 ounces almonds

4.5 ounces pecans

1 cup plus 2 tablespoons brown rice flour or buckwheat flour, plus more to dust

6 tablespoons maple syrup

2 tablespoons ground ginger

1 tablespoon coconut oil, plus more for the baking sheets (optional)

1 tablespoon chia seeds

Preheat the oven to 400°F (convection 350°F).

Place the almonds and pecans in a food processor and blend for 1 minute or so until a flour forms. Then add all the other ingredients, pour in 6 tablespoons of water and blend into a sticky dough mixture.

Get a couple of baking sheets ready, either oiling them with coconut oil or lining them with parchment paper.

Dust a work surface and a rolling pin with flour and roll the dough out until it's ¼ inch thick and perfectly smooth. At this point, use your chosen cookie cutter to cut out the cookies, then put them on the prepared baking sheets.

Bake for 15–20 minutes, until golden, then leave to cool on the baking sheet before storing in an airtight container. They will keep for up to 5 days.

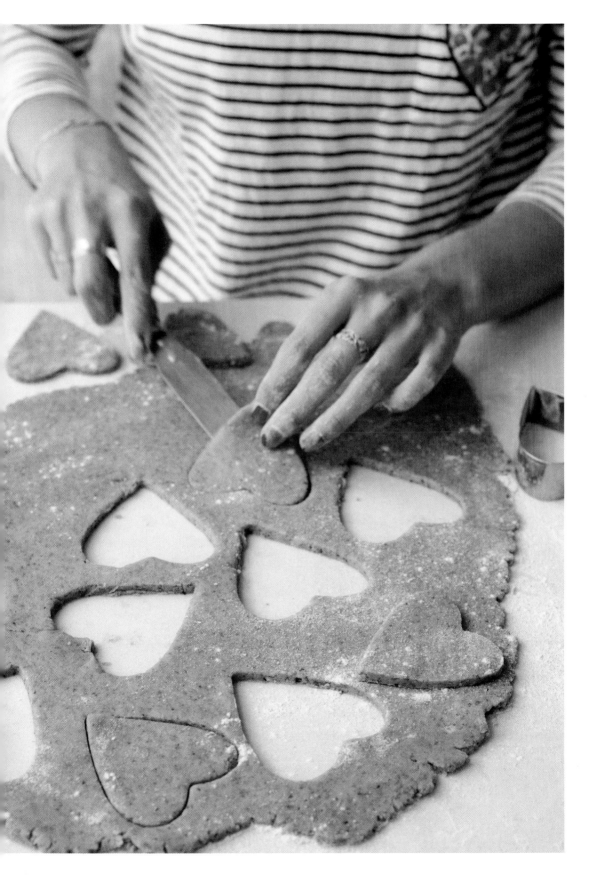

These have been a staple in my house for the last few years. They're the easiest snack to travel with and they last for a good three weeks, so you can make a big batch and keep them in the fridge to ensure that you have a delicious pick-me-up when you need one. The lime and ginger version is sharper and tangier, which is so refreshing; the cinnamon and honey variety is richer, more like a dessert. They both have the same base, so I often make a little of each, so I have a mix of flavors to choose from when I'm hungry.

ENERGY BITES, TWO WAYS

Each makes 15

LIME AND GINGER

4.5 ounces cashews
large handful of pumpkin seeds
I tablespoon chia seeds
7 ounces medjool dates, pitted
juice of I lime
I tablespoon ground ginger

Place the cashews, pumpkin seeds and chia seeds into a food processor and blend for 30 seconds, until the nuts and seeds are crushed but have not yet become a flour.

Add the dates to the mixture with the lime juice and ground ginger and blend until it becomes nice and sticky.

Scoop 2 teaspoons of the mixture into your hand and roll it into a ball. Repeat until all the mixture has been used up.

Place the bites in the freezer for I hour to set, then store in the fridge.

CINNAMON AND HONEY

4.5 ounces cashews
large handful of pumpkin seeds
I tablespoon chia seeds
3.5 ounces medjool dates, pitted
I tablespoon honey
2 teaspoons almond butter
4 teaspoons ground cinnamon

Place the cashews, pumpkin seeds and chia seeds into a food processor and blend for 30 seconds, until the nuts and seeds are crushed but have not yet become a flour.

Add the dates to the mixture with the honey, almond butter and cinnamon and blend until it becomes nice and sticky.

Make and store the bites as before (at left).

The cookies I make when I'm home and need something to nibble on but don't want to start making a big mess in the kitchen. They only use one bowl and one baking sheet so they're very fuss-free and there's absolutely no chopping required: all you have to do is throw the ingredients together, then bake them. I love eating these with a layer of almond or cashew butter spread on top for extra deliciousness. The cacao nibs add a marvelous chocolatey crunch.

CACAO, OAT AND RAISIN COOKIES

Makes 16

1¾ cups plus 2 tablespoons
   rolled oats
generous ½ cup raisins
½ cup almond-meal
generous ¾ cup Apple Purée
   (page 40)
6 tablespoons date syrup
1 tablespoon tahini
1 tablespoon raw cacao powder
1.75 ounces cacao nibs

Preheat the oven to 340°F (convection 300°F).

Simply place all the ingredients into a bowl and stir them together until a sticky mixture forms.

Line a baking sheet with parchment paper.

Scoop 1 tablespoon of the mixture into your hand and roll it into a ball. Place the ball on the baking sheet and squish it down so the bottom is flat, but keep the middle of the cookie about ¾ inch thick.

Repeat to form 16 cookies, then place the baking sheet in the oven to bake for 20 minutes.

Let the cookies cool on the pan, then store them in an airtight container. They will keep for up to 5 days.

Tweak It

Try adding dried cranberries to these if you have some lying around, they add a delicious flavor and a great pop of color. Substitute them for some of the raisins, using about ¼ cup of each.

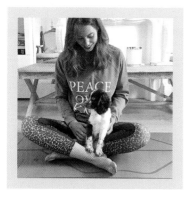

I have to admit something here: the second time I made these, I never actually assembled the treats, instead I poured everything into a bowl and ate it in front of a movie. Be warned, you'll probably want to do the same thing! They're the best little treat, though, as they only need five ingredients and they take just five minutes to make and ten minutes to set, so you can have a sweet dessert or snack in just fifteen minutes. They don't taste at all healthy either; instead totally rich, chocolatey and indulgent. You'll need mini muffin liners for these.

QUINOA AND CACAO CRISPY TREATS

Makes 20

5 tablespoons coconut oil

½ cup plus 2 tablespoons raw cacao powder

6 tablespoons maple syrup

2 tablespoons almond butter, or any other nut butter

4 cups popped/puffed quinoa

Place the coconut oil, cacao powder, maple syrup and almond butter into a saucepan and gently heat it for a few minutes until it is totally smooth and melted.

Meanwhile, pour the quinoa pops into a mixing bowl.

Once the mixture has melted, pour it over the quinoa pops and stir it together until all the quinoa is covered in chocolate.

Scoop the mixture into mini muffin liners and place in the freezer for about 10 minutes, until totally stuck together.

Shop Sense

If you're not sure where to buy quinoa pops/puffed quinoa, then just have a look online; it's always available!

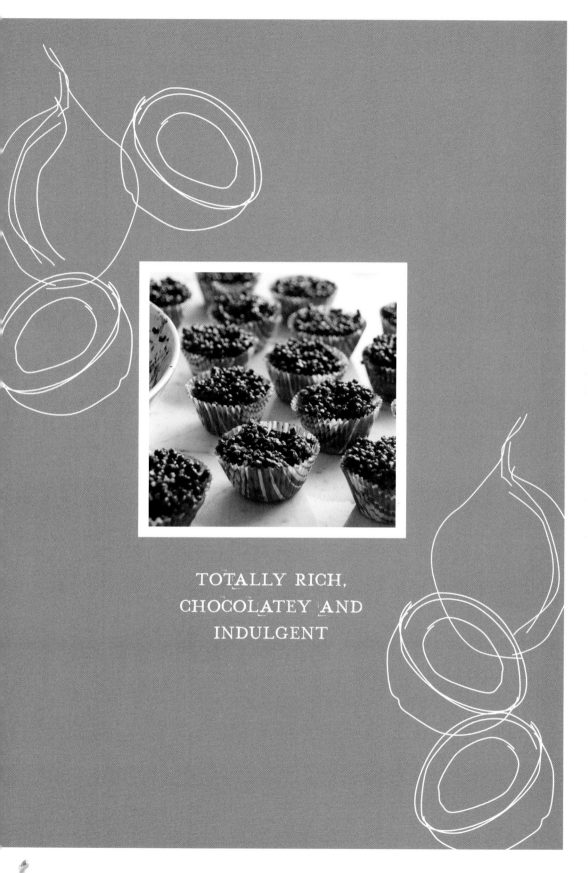

TOTALLY RICH,
CHOCOLATEY AND
INDULGENT

This is my go-to snack when I'm traveling or have busy days. I love keeping a jar of it on my desk so I can pick at it throughout the day to keep my energy levels high. I use a mix of Brazil nuts, hazelnuts and cashews, but all nuts are delicious here: blanched almonds, pecans and walnuts are great, too.

TRAIL MIX, TWO WAYS

Both make 1 big jar

CINNAMON AND MAPLE

3.5 ounces Brazil nuts

5 ounces blanched hazelnuts

7 ounces cashews

3 tablespoons maple syrup

½ teaspoon ground cinnamon

salt

1¼ cups raisins

Preheat the oven to 425°F (convection 400°F).

Spread the nuts on a large baking sheet and add the maple syrup, cinnamon and a sprinkling of salt. Stir everything together.

Place the baking sheet in the oven for 10 minutes, then take it out and stir everything before returning it to the oven for another 10 minutes.

Take out of the oven and stir in the raisins.

Leave until cooled, then store in an airtight jar.

CHILI AND TAMARI

3.5 ounces Brazil nuts

5 ounces blanched hazelnuts

7 ounces cashews

4 teaspoons tamari

1 tablespoon olive oil

1 teaspoon chili flakes

salt

Preheat the oven to 425°F (convection 400°F).

Spread the nuts on a large baking sheet and add the tamari, olive oil, chili flakes and a sprinkling of salt. Stir everything together.

Place the baking sheet in the oven for 10 minutes, then take it out and stir everything before returning it to the oven for another 10 minutes.

Leave until cooled, then store in an airtight jar.

Kitchen Know-How

Make sure to use a big baking sheet, so that none of the nuts have to sit on top of each other. This stops them from going soggy.

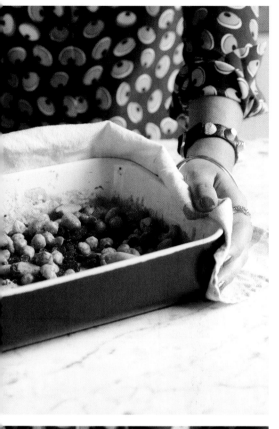
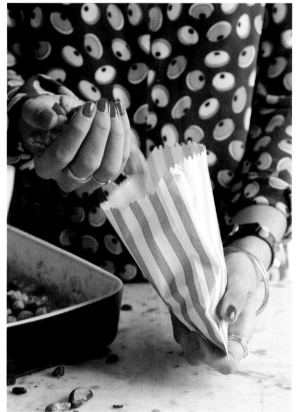
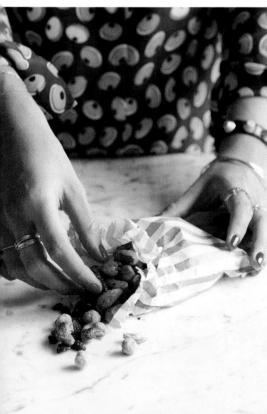
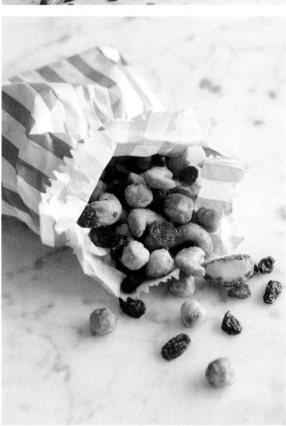

This is so much fun. I just love waiting for the corn to pop and then hearing the sound of all the kernels hitting the roof of the pan. It's pretty satisfying popping your own corn, too, rather than putting a bag in the microwave! The popcorn topping is so dreamy—a mix of coconut oil with coconut sugar, fresh vanilla and cinnamon—which together tastes so perfect!

CINNAMON-COCONUT POPCORN

Makes 1 big bowl

4 tablespoons coconut oil
scant ½ cup popcorn kernels
3 tablespoons coconut sugar
2 teaspoons vanilla powder
2 teaspoons ground cinnamon

Put 1 tablespoon of coconut oil in a saucepan with only about 3 kernels of popcorn. Place the lid on the saucepan and set over medium-high heat until the kernels pop.

Once the kernels have popped, remove them from the pan and add all the other kernels, making sure to put the lid on! Let them cook until they all pop.

While you wait, melt the remaining 3 tablespoons of coconut oil in a saucepan over medium-low heat. Once it has melted, stir in the coconut sugar, vanilla and cinnamon.

Pour the mixture over the popcorn once it has all popped and stir well to coat.

Kitchen Know-How

Be patient while you make the recipe, the kernels always take a bit longer to pop than you expect!

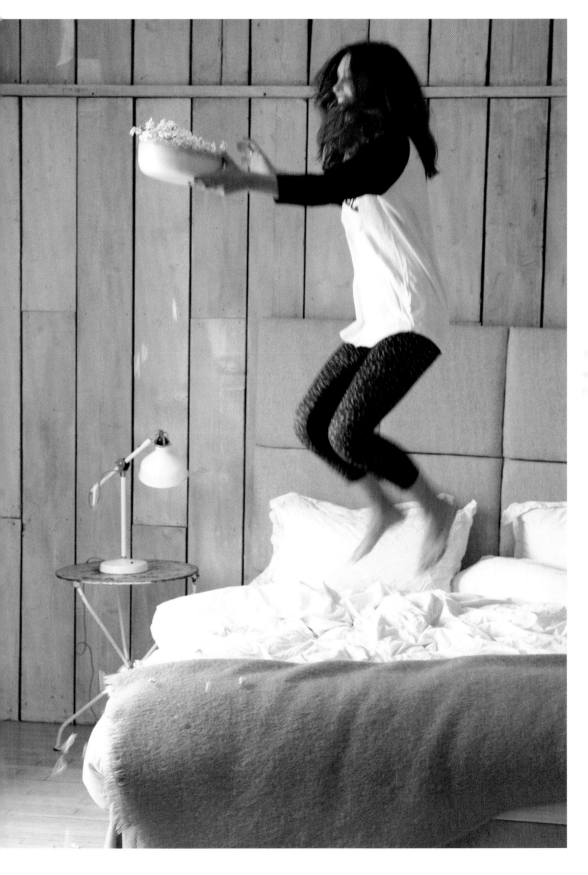

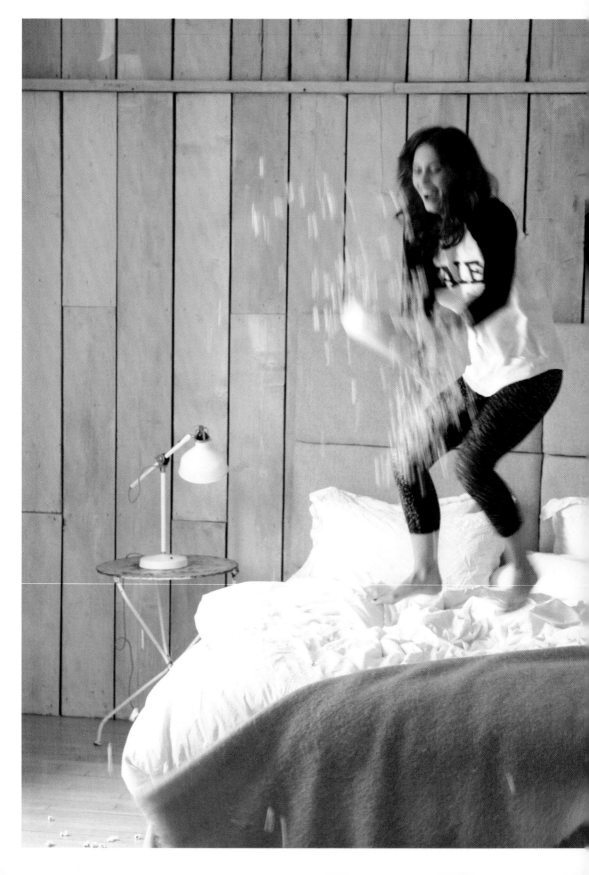

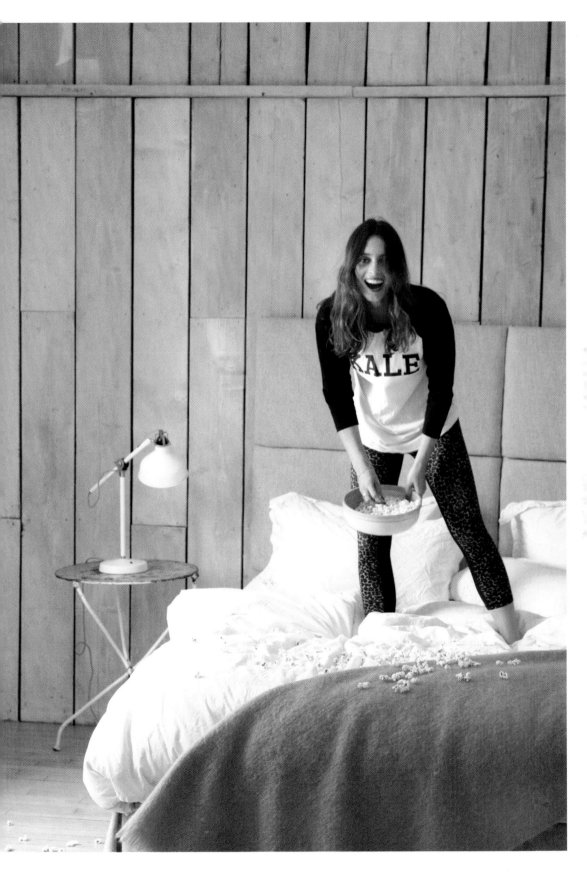

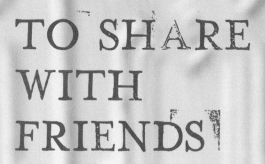

TO SHARE WITH FRIENDS

The best desserts for
showing off and chilling out

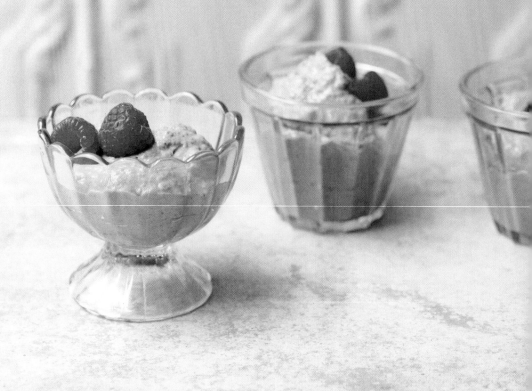

Such a good option if you need a five-minute dessert for friends. They really only take that long to make, but the end result is so delicious that you'll delight everyone at the table! The mix of coconut, almond butter and avocado means the mousse is rich and creamy, while the raspberries add a subtle sharpness that the honey and vanilla balance out perfectly. I love serving these in little glasses with extra raspberries and a drizzling of honey on top, it makes them look and taste beautiful.

COCONUT AND RASPBERRY MOUSSE

Serves 6

3.5 ounces solid coconut cream (in a block)

1 avocado

1 vanilla pod

3 tablespoons almond butter

1 pound raspberries, plus more to serve (optional)

2 tablespoons honey, plus more to serve (optional)

Chop the block of coconut cream into quarters and place in a food processor. Scoop the avocado flesh out of the skin and into the processor. Scrape the vanilla seeds out of the pod into the processor.

Add all the remaining ingredients and blend until a smooth, rich mousse forms.

Spoon it into 6 glasses and place in the fridge for 1 hour to set before serving, with more raspberries and a drizzle of honey, if you like.

The best summer dessert. It's such a crowd pleaser, as it doesn't look or taste scary and healthy, but is full of goodness. I love using strawberries and banana slices for the fruit layer as they're so sweet and together have an almost creamy texture, while the cacao- and vanilla-infused oaty topping adds a crunchiness to each bite, which perfectly contrasts with the fruit. The other great thing about this recipe is that it requires no equipment, very little washing up or chopping and it only takes five to ten minutes of preparation; so it's great if you're short on time but still need to create something delicious!

SUMMER STRAWBERRY-BANANA CRUMBLE

Serves 6 – 8

8 bananas
1 pint strawberries
8 tablespoons maple syrup
3¾ cups rolled oats
1½ cups almond-meal
2 teaspoons raw cacao powder
1 teaspoon vanilla powder
¼ cup coconut oil
1 teaspoon ground cinnamon

Preheat the oven to 400°F (convection 350°F).

Slice the bananas into a bowl, then chop the strawberries into bite-size pieces and mix them in with the bananas.

Place the fruit in a baking dish (mine is 12 x 8 inches) and drizzle 2 tablespoons of the maple syrup over them. Put the dish in the oven to bake for 10 minutes.

Meanwhile, make the crumble layer. Add all the remaining ingredients, except the coconut oil and cinnamon, to a mixing bowl, not forgetting the rest of the maple syrup.

Put the coconut oil in a saucepan with the cinnamon on low heat until it's melted, then pour into the bowl and mix all the ingredients together.

Once the fruit has cooked for 10 minutes, take the baking dish out of the oven and spread the crumble layer over the top.

Place the dish back in the oven and cook for 20 minutes, until the top turns a golden brown.

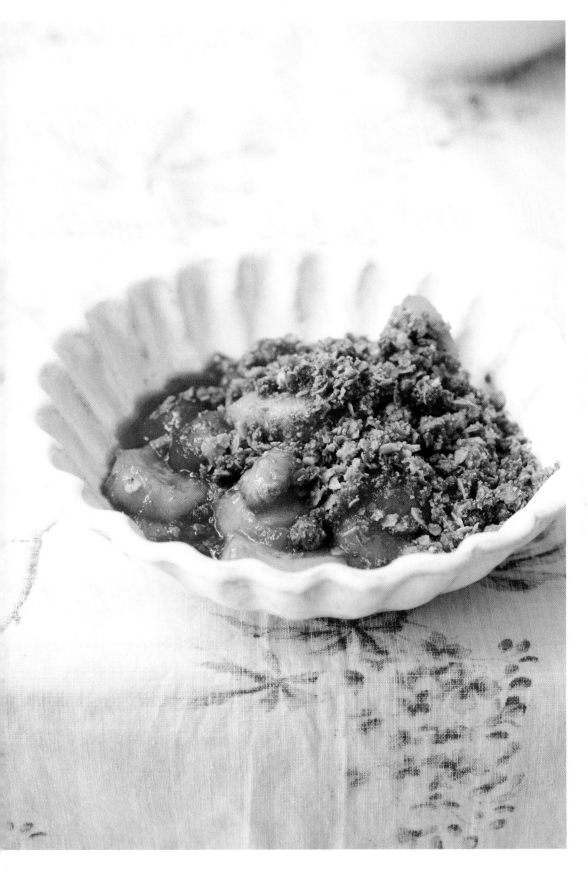

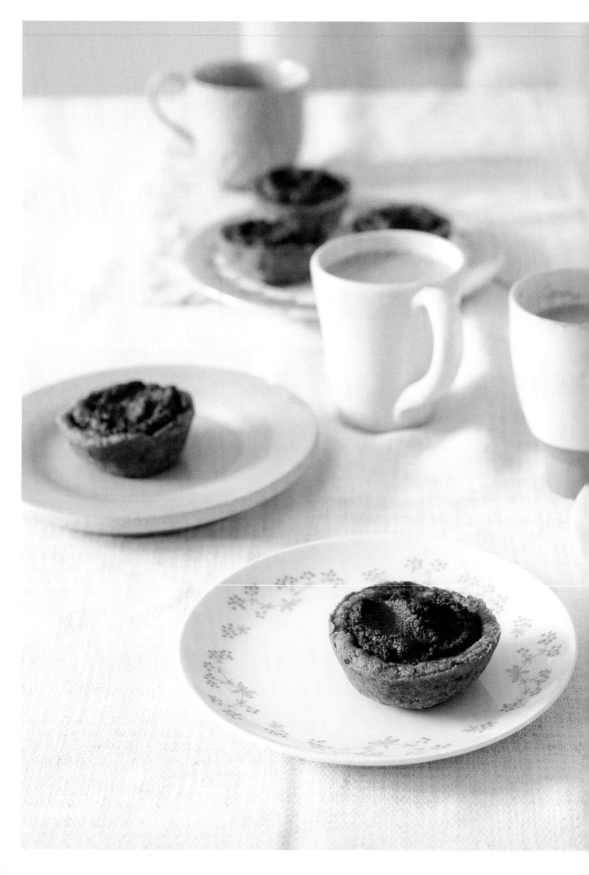

These are divine, a dream dessert. Nothing about them really looks or tastes healthy, but somehow I managed to sneak some avocado into them. They are great to serve to friends as they'll impress everyone.

CHOCOLATE AND HAZELNUT TARTS

Makes 12

For the filling

5 ounces hazelnuts (generous 1 cup)
¾ cup maple syrup
¼ cup raw cacao powder
1 avocado, peeled and pitted
pinch of salt

For the base

14 medjool dates, pitted
3 cups plus 3 tablespoons almond-meal
¼ cup coconut oil, plus more for the tin
brown rice flour or buckwheat flour, to dust

Preheat the oven to 350°F (convection 325°F).

Place the hazelnuts on a baking sheet and put in the oven to roast for 10 minutes. Remove and allow to cool. (Leave the oven on.)

Meanwhile, make the base. Place all the ingredients except the flour into a food processor along with 3 tablespoons of water and blend until a sticky mixture forms.

Sprinkle a little flour on a work surface and roll the mixture out.

Use a little coconut oil to oil 12 cups of a muffin tin.

Using a cookie cutter, a saucer or whatever you can find, cut rounds of the base mixture a little wider than each muffin shape, then mold the dough rounds into the muffin cups.

Put the bases in the oven to cook for 10–15 minutes, until they turn a golden brown. Remove and allow to cool.

Once the hazelnuts are cool, place them in a blender and blend until they form a nut butter, then add the remaining filling ingredients with 7 tablespoons of water.

When the bases are completely cool (this is important as it lets them harden and stops the chocolate from melting), fill each one with a generous tablespoon of the filling.

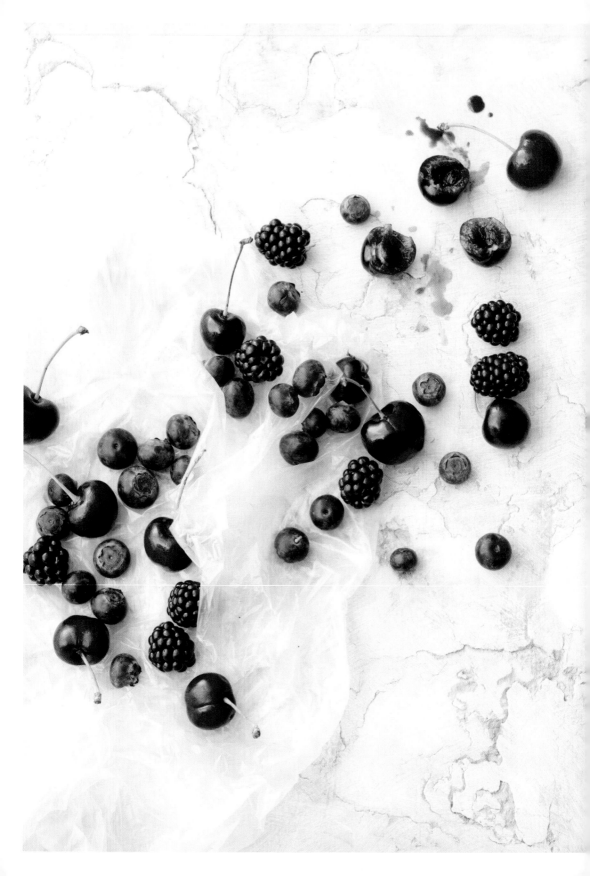

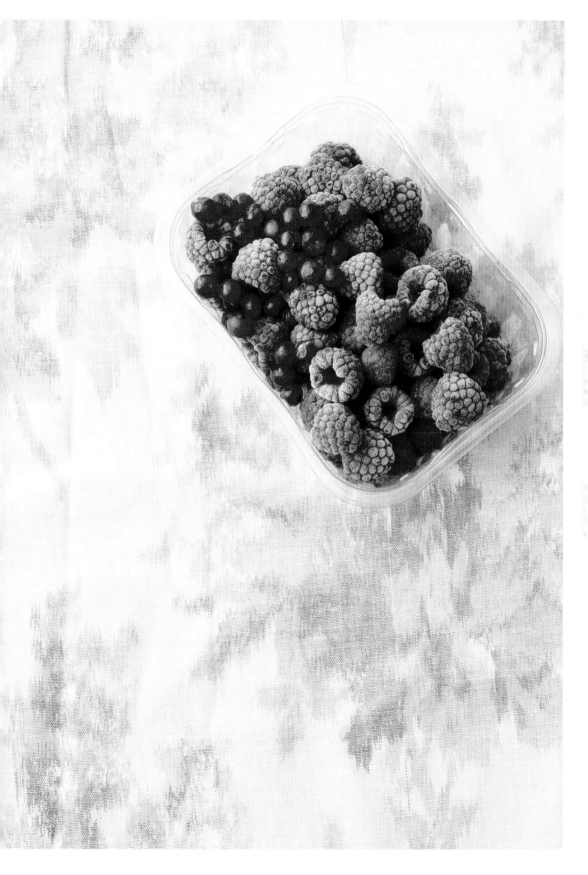

The idea for this crumble came from my new-found love of mince pies! Last winter, my brother and I wanted to make a mince pie–inspired, Christmassy dessert for my family and this was the result . . . it was such a hit that I just had to share it with you all. The mix of apples, pears, raisins and spices is so warming and delicious, while the spiced crumble topping is bursting with wonderful flavors and crunchy textures that complement the fruit perfectly.

WINTER-SPICED PEAR AND APPLE CRUMBLE

Serves 6–8

For the fruit layer

5 red apples

3 pears

I teaspoon ground cinnamon

I teaspoon ground ginger

generous ¾ cup raisins

For the crumble layer

7 ounces pecans (about 2 cups)

3¾ cups rolled oats

2 teaspoons vanilla powder

¼ cup coconut oil

½ cup date syrup

2 teaspoons ground ginger

2 teaspoons ground cinnamon

coconut yogurt, to serve
    (optional)

Start by making the fruit layer. Peel and core the apples and pears, then chop them into bite-size pieces.

Place the chopped pieces into a saucepan with the cinnamon, ginger and raisins, plus enough water to cover the bottom inch or so of the pan. Let the fruit gently cook over medium-low heat for about 20 minutes, until it's really soft.

Preheat the oven to 400°F (convection 350°F).

Meanwhile, make the crumble layer. Process the pecans in a food processor for about 30 seconds, until they form a flour. Tip into a bowl and mix in the oats and vanilla.

Place the coconut oil, date syrup, ginger and cinnamon in a saucepan and gently heat the mixture until the coconut oil melts. Pour this into the oat mixture and stir it all together.

Once the fruit has cooked, place it in a baking dish (mine is 12 x 8 inches) and spread the crumble layer on top. Bake for 20 minutes, until the top turns a golden brown. Serve with coconut yogurt, if you like.

Make It Better

If you want to create something extra-indulgent, then try drizzling maple syrup across the top of the crumble once it has finished baking. It makes it extra-sweet and delicious!

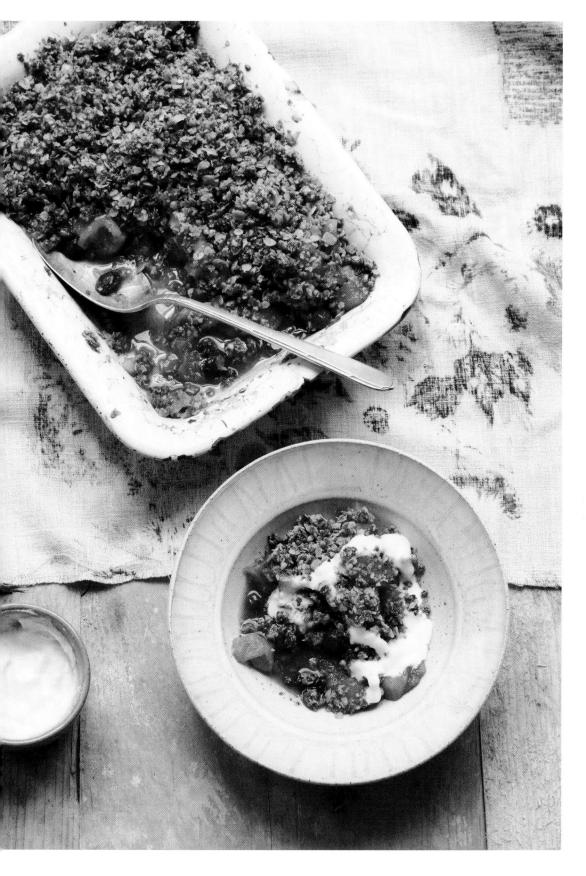

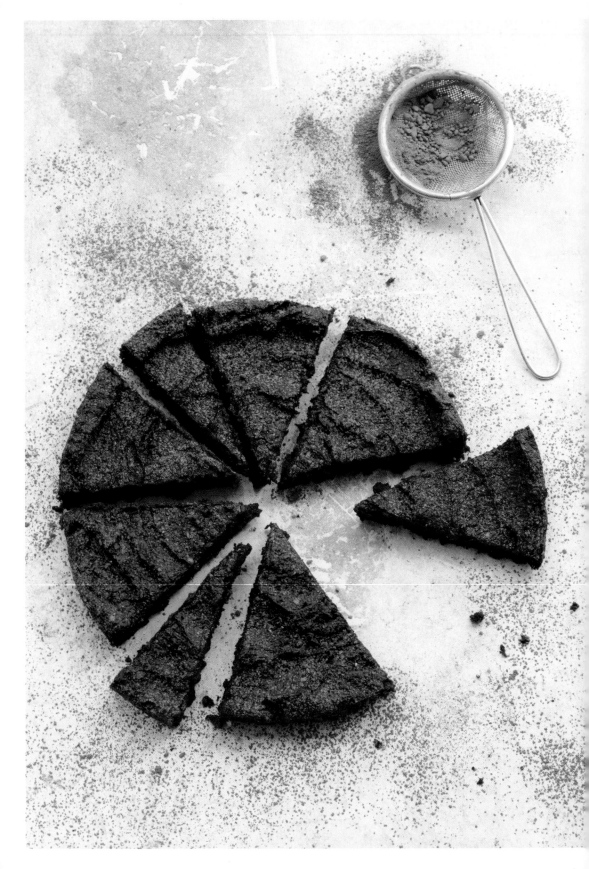

My favorite chocolate cake, it's just so soft and gooey. It may also be the simplest cake ever: just six ingredients blended together and then baked for thirty minutes, so it's great if you need a fancy dessert but have limited time or energy! It's perfect for a party, too, as I've yet to find anyone who doesn't love it.

CHOCOLATE GANACHE CAKE

Makes 1 cake

For the cake

coconut oil, for the pan

3 avocados

7 tablespoons almond butter

½ cup raw cacao powder, plus more to dust (optional)

1½ cups plus 3 tablespoons maple syrup

1½ cups almond-meal

3 tablespoons chia seeds

For the frosting

¼ cup coconut oil

¼ cup raw cacao powder

¼ cup maple syrup

Preheat the oven to 350°F (convection 325°F). Oil an 8-inch cake pan with coconut oil; I don't line it with parchment paper as I use a silicone pan. If yours isn't, you might want to.

Scoop the avocado flesh out of the skins and into a food processor. Add all the other ingredients and blend until smooth. Scrape the batter into the prepared pan and level the top.

Bake for 30 minutes, or until a knife inserted into the center comes out clean. Leave to cool and bind together for at least 20 minutes before turning out of the pan.

Sift over a little more cacao powder, if you like, to serve, as we did for the photo, or make the frosting. For the frosting, warm the coconut oil in a small saucepan just until it melts. Stir in all the other ingredients until you have a smooth, glossy glaze. Use it to frost the top of the cooled cake, then leave to set.

Make It Better

This cake is perfect just as it is, frosted or not, but you could add a scoop of coconut ice cream to each slice if you want.

A great dessert to serve to friends. It tastes incredibly caramel-like, but it's full of goodness. The middle layer is my favorite part, as the amazing combination of pecans, cashew butter, dates and maple syrup is so heavenly, especially with the maple-roasted pecans arranged on top.

PECAN PIE

Makes 1 pie

For the crust

5 ounces almonds (about 1 cup)
1 cup buckwheat flour
2 teaspoons ground cinnamon
2 tablespoons honey
4 medjool dates, pitted
2 tablespoons coconut oil, plus more for the dish

For the middle

4.5 ounces pecans (about 1¼ cups)
10 tablespoons cashew butter
¼ cup maple syrup
12 medjool dates, pitted

For the topping

1¼ cup pecans
2 tablespoons maple syrup
1 teaspoon ground cinnamon

Preheat the oven to 400°F (convection 350°F).

Make the crust. Place the almonds into a food processor and grind to a flour, then add the buckwheat flour, cinnamon, honey, dates and coconut oil and blend to a sticky mixture.

Oil a pie dish, then cover the bottom with the crust. Bake for about 15 minutes, until it becomes nicely browned and is hardening.

Meanwhile, make the middle layer. First place the pecans in the food processor for a minute to crush them into a cross between a nut butter and a flour, then add the cashew butter. Once those have mixed, add the maple syrup and dates. Allow these to blend as you gradually add ¾ cup of water. Keep this in the fridge until you're ready to spread it over the base.

Finally, place the pecans for the topping on a baking sheet with the maple syrup and cinnamon, mix them together and bake for 5 minutes, until a little browned and crunchy.

Once the pie base has cooked, allow it to sit for a few minutes before spreading the middle layer across it and adding the pecans on top. Leave it for 1 hour or so to set fully.

Tweak It

Sadly, if you're allergic to nuts, this dessert isn't for you; the pecans are just too essential! If you can't eat almonds, though, try switching those for any other nut, while the cashew butter can be switched for almond butter or Brazil nut butter.

So incredibly rich, creamy and indulgent, you'd never know there was anything healthy in there. The nutty bottom layer is wonderfully thick and almost chewy, while the top tastes gooey, just like cheesecake. The magic ingredient for this is avocado, which sounds crazy but trust me: the flavor disappears beneath the chocolatey goodness and you're left with just its divine texture, plus all the wonderful life-giving health properties.

DOUBLE-CHOCOLATE CHEESECAKE BROWNIES

Makes 16

For the brownie layer

14 ounces medjool dates, pitted
5 ounces pecans (about
   1¼ cups), plus a few more,
   chopped, for the top (optional)
2.5 ounces almonds (about
   ½ cup)
2 tablespoons raw cacao powder

For the cheesecake layer

2 large or 3 small avocados,
   peeled and pitted
1 ripe banana
5 ounces medjool dates, pitted
3 tablespoons maple syrup
3 tablespoons raw cacao powder
2 tablespoons almond butter

Start with the brownie layer. Place all the ingredients into a food processor. Blend for 2–3 minutes until the mixture becomes nice and sticky, but still with some little nutty pieces, as they create a deliciously crunchy texture.

Place the brownie mixture into a deep baking tray lined with parchment paper, using a spatula to press it down firmly. Set aside.

To make the cheesecake layer, simply place all the ingredients into the food processor and blend until a really creamy, chocolatey custard-like deliciousness forms! This should take 5 minutes, depending on the strength of your processor.

Pour this mixture over the brownie base. You can then sprinkle a few pecan pieces on the top, if you want. Place the whole thing in the freezer and freeze for about 2 hours. Remove from the freezer 10 minutes before you want to slice and serve the brownies. Cut into 16 brownies to serve.

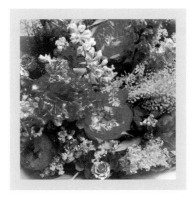

One of the pricier recipes in the book, as it's very nut-heavy, but trust me, it is such a treat. The three layers melt together perfectly like little bites of paradise, with the ideal mix of cookie, caramel and chocolate, just like a super-healthy, even-more-delicious version of millionaire's shortbread.

CHOCOLATE CARAMEL SLICES

Makes about 16

For the base

5 ounces almonds (about 1 cup)
5 ounces pecans (about 1¼ cups)
14 ounces medjool dates, pitted
2 tablespoons almond butter

For the caramel layer

14 ounces medjool dates, pitted
6 heaping tablespoons
   almond butter
2 tablespoons maple syrup
1 teaspoon coconut oil

For the chocolate layer

3.5 ounces cacao butter
1 tablespoon almond butter
5 ounces medjool dates, pitted
2 tablespoons raw cacao powder
2–4 tablespoons maple syrup
   (depending on how sweet you
   like it)

Start by making the base: simply put the almonds and pecans in a food processor and blend for about 1 minute until a grainy flour forms, then add the dates and almond butter and blend again until the mixture becomes nice and sticky. Transfer the mixture to the bottom of a baking pan lined with parchment paper (mine is 12 x 8 x 2 inches), pushing it down firmly with a spatula. Place the pan in the freezer for 20 minutes.

Next make the caramel layer. To do this simply put all the ingredients into the food processor with ½ cup of water and blend until smooth and creamy, then pour onto the base layer and put the pan back into the freezer for 30–40 minutes, so it becomes firm enough to pour on the chocolate layer.

Finally make the chocolate layer. Place the cacao butter and the almond butter in a saucepan and melt on a low heat. Once they've melted, pour into the food processor with the remaining ingredients and blend until smooth.

After the caramel has become solid, spread the chocolate layer on top, then place the pan back into the freezer for about 2 hours.

Take them out and leave at room temperature for 15–20 minutes, to let them warm up a little, then cut them into 16 slices to serve.

Nut-Free?

Sadly there's no nut replacement here, so I'm afraid if you can't have any nuts this isn't for you. If you're simply allergic to almonds or pecans, then substitute them with cashews or hazelnuts, and cashew butter.

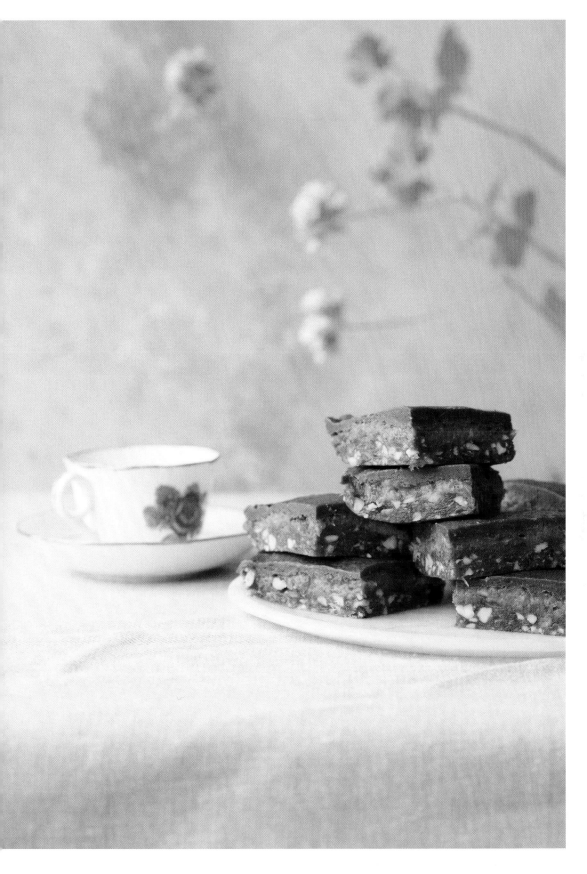

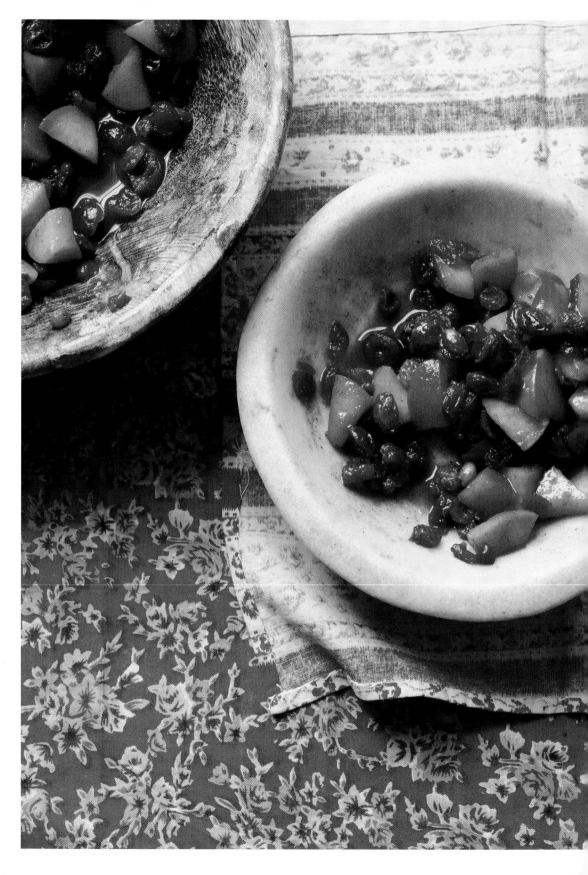

This dish was inspired by the mixture I made for mince pies last Christmas. I loved the mincemeat combination so much that I started making big batches of it to eat as an easy dessert when I wanted something light and easy. Each bite has a beautiful rich flavor thanks to the blend of dried fruits, vanilla, cinnamon and ginger, which together tastes so amazing. I often eat this just as it is, but it's especially delicious served with coconut yogurt or coconut ice cream.

SPICED FRUIT BOWLS

Serves 6

6 red apples
2 vanilla pods
juice of 4 oranges
3.5 ounces dried cranberries
1¼ cups golden raisins
1¼ cups raisins
2 tablespoons coconut oil
2 tablespoons date syrup
2 teaspoons ground ginger
2 teaspoons ground cinnamon

Core the apples, chop into small pieces and place them into a saucepan.

Slice the vanilla pods in half and scrape the seeds into the pan.

Add all the remaining ingredients and stir it together. Let it simmer over a gentle heat for about 40 minutes, until the apples are nice and soft.

Serve and enjoy.

Make It Better

I love making extra of this so that I can keep it in the fridge and add it to my porridge in the morning, it's so delicious!

Inspired by some truffles I was sent and loved so much that I spent days trying to re-create them! They're similar to the chocolate energy bites from my blog that are so popular; but these are much creamier and softer in the middle, with chunks of crunchy nuts and a layer of baobab powder on the outside, which is what gives them a great taste. Baobab is the most amazing source of vitamin C, too, so these truffles are just what you need when you're feeling run-down.

BAOBAB TRUFFLES

Makes 15–20

17 ounces medjool dates, pitted

7 ounces almonds (about 1¼ cups)

¼ cup coconut oil

¼ cup raw cacao powder

2 tablespoons almond butter

5 tablespoons baobab powder

Place everything, except the baobab powder, in a food processor and blend the mixture until it has stuck together, but the nuts are still in chunks.

Place the baobab powder in a bowl.

Scoop 1 tablespoon of truffle mixture and roll it into a ball, then roll it in the baobab powder so it's coated and no longer sticky. Repeat to coat all the balls.

Place in the fridge for a few hours to set, then serve.

Tweak It

If you don't have any baobab, then try rolling the truffles in more raw cacao powder instead, for an extra-chocolatey bite.

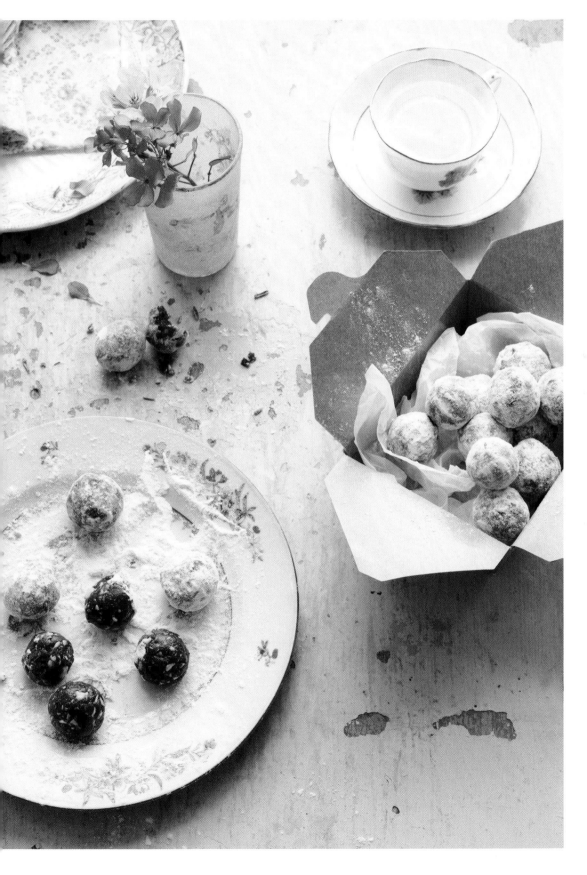

SOOTHING DRINKS

For warming, calming, cleansing
and just adoring: hugs in mugs

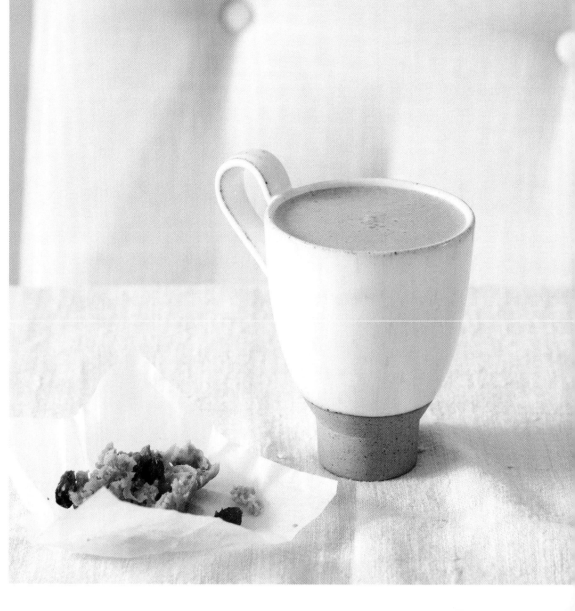

Just so simple and delicious. This is great if you're craving something sweet after a meal and don't want to make or eat a big dessert. I drink it all winter, as it really warms you up from the inside out, like a giant hug in a mug.

HOT CHOCOLATE

Serves 1

1 cup plant-based milk
  (homemade is best here)
2 tablespoons date syrup
2 teaspoons raw cacao powder
1 teaspoon almond butter

Place all the ingredients into a saucepan and heat gently. Keep stirring as the hot chocolate heats, to ensure all the ingredients mix together and the almond butter doesn't sink and stick to the bottom.

Take the pan off the heat before it reaches the boiling point, to keep all the goodness in.

Make It Better

If you're feeling indulgent, use coconut milk in this recipe for the sweetest, creamiest hot chocolate ever.

I know the idea of a warm beet juice may sound strange, but this is one of those recipes where you just have to trust me that the outcome is amazing and you won't find it weird at all as you enjoy it. When I first created this recipe I honestly thought it was revolutionary, as it's the perfect drink when you need something to warm you up. It's lighter than Hot Chocolate (page 235) but still nicely sweet, perfect for an afternoon tonic on a cold day.

WARM BEET AND APPLE JUICE

Serves 1

1 beet
3 carrots
2 apples

Simply peel the beet, then put it through a juicer with the carrots and apples. Pour the juice into a saucepan.

Gently heat the saucepan for a couple of minutes, keeping it over low heat at all times; you want it to cook slowly. Take it off the heat before it comes to a boil.

Once the juice is nice and warm, but not boiling hot, pour it into a mug and enjoy!

Kitchen Know-How

Don't try adding greens to this; trust me, it's really not nice! Instead, if you want a green kick, have a separate green juice or smoothie.

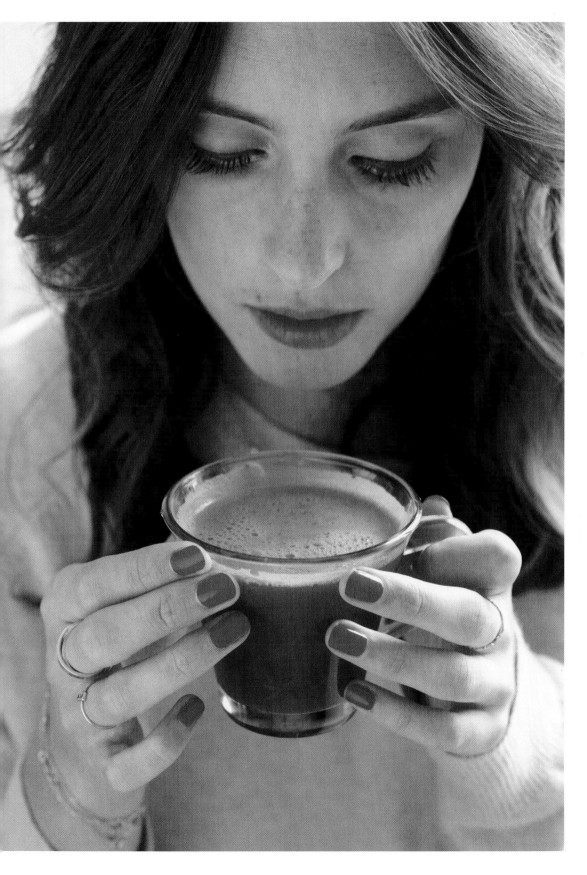

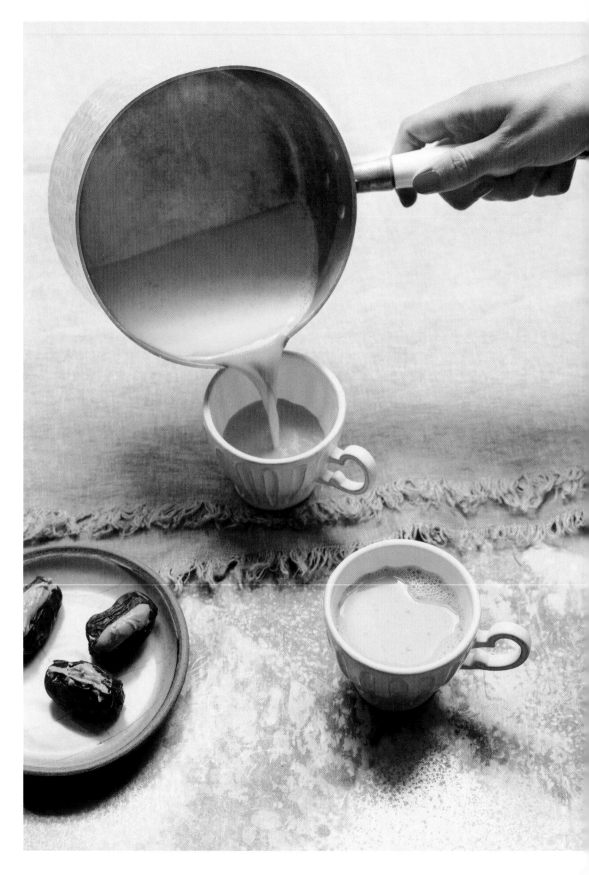

The most soothing bedtime drink. Each delicious sip will calm your mind and body down, leaving you feeling amazing and very relaxed. The blend of cashew milk, honey and turmeric is wonderfully balanced, while the turmeric adds a warming touch. I love drinking a big mug of this when I'm feeling tired and run-down, or just before I go to bed to help me ease into a deep sleep.

WARMING TURMERIC TONIC

Serves 1

1 cup cashew milk (for
   homemade, see page 53)
1 heaping teaspoon honey
1 teaspoon ground turmeric

Place the cashew milk in a saucepan and allow it to heat gently; it should take about 2 minutes to get hot enough to drink. Don't let it come to a boil, to preserve the nutrients.

Once the milk is hot, stir in the honey and turmeric and let it all infuse together for a couple of seconds.

Pour the drink into a mug.

Tweak It

If you don't have any turmeric—or you're not a big fan of the spice—try adding a little ground ginger instead, or simply enjoy the sweet mix of cashew milk and honey on its own.

If you're feeling in need of a sweet
tonic, a big mug of this tea is exactly
what you want. It's also great if you want
something rounded and flavorsome,
but you're not really hungry enough for
dessert. The honey makes it deliciously
sweet, while the lemon gives a citrus
infusion and the ginger and cayenne work
to add a touch of spice to each sip.

One of my favorite things in the world.
As a family, we're all obsessed with mint
tea and have it all the time after dinner.
It's such a soothing, comforting drink
that feels so good after a big meal! The
mint is calming on the stomach and it has
a delicious flavor that sates a mild sweet
craving, which is perfect if you're trying to
cut back on sugar!

SPICY HONEY LEMON TEA

Serves 1

scant 1 ounce fresh ginger
juice of ¼ lemon
pinch of cayenne pepper
1–2 teaspoons honey

Peel the ginger, then cut it into 4 chunks
and place these in a saucepan with 1¼ cups of
water. Let it boil for about 10 minutes.

Pour the water from the saucepan into a
mug, leaving the chunks of ginger behind.

Stir in the lemon juice, cayenne and honey.

Tweak It

If you don't like things too hot, omit the
cayenne pepper; the ginger will be spicy
enough on its own.

FRESH MINT TEA

Serves 1

3.5 ounces fresh mint leaves

Place the mint leaves in a teapot with
6 cups of boiling water and let it sit for 15
minutes, so that the mint flavor infuses into
the water.

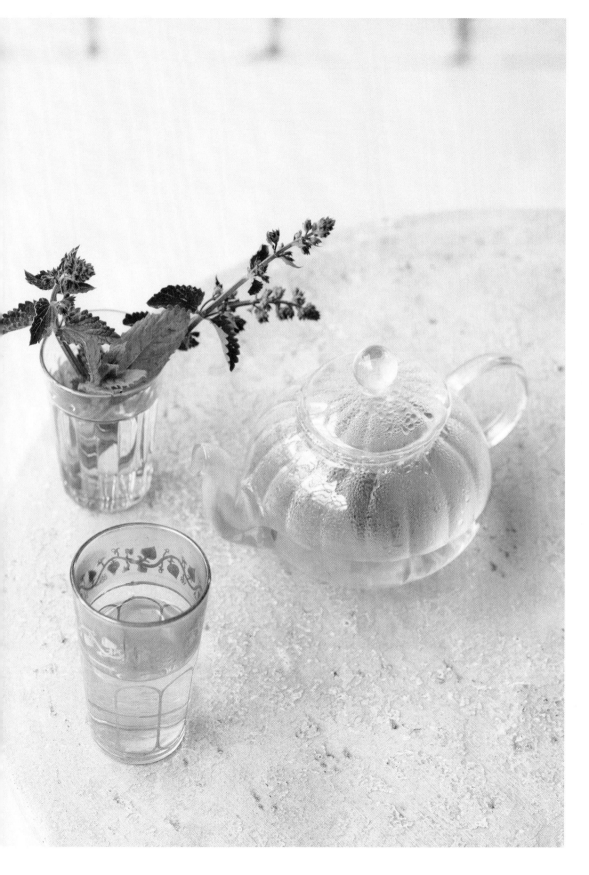

RECIPE INDEX

INDEX

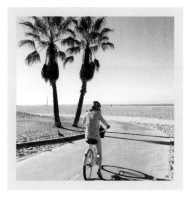

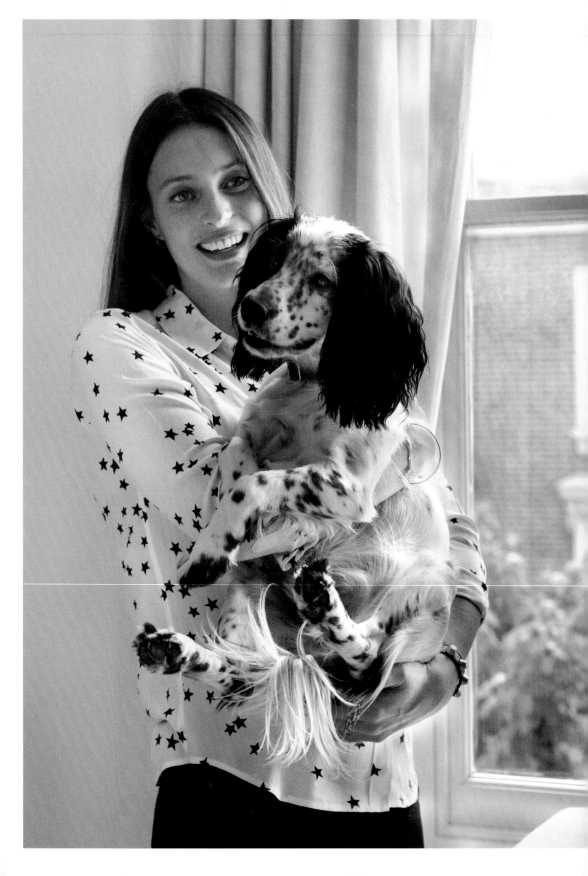

THANK YOU

I'm so excited to have had the opportunity to write a second book. I've absolutely loved the experience and I feel like the luckiest person in the world to be able to do this as a career, but I'd never have managed it without all of you, so I wanted to take a minute to thank a lot of people in my life.

More than anything, I am so grateful for the support of everyone who reads and follows Deliciously Ella. I'm continually overwhelmed by how many of you love what I do, it's absolutely crazy and so incredible. I can't believe how much this community has grown since I started blogging and it's so exciting to see more and more people become interested in healthy living. So thank you all for spreading the healthy happy message and for supporting Deliciously Ella: I appreciate each message you send and every photo you share. You're so inspiring.

Thank you to my family, for being so supportive of everything I do. You've given me amazing love and guidance with everything in my life, but your constant encouragement of Deliciously Ella is just so awesome. You've instilled so much confidence in me to pursue what I'm passionate about and I'm so grateful for that.

Thank you to my amazing friends Annie and Livia. You have saved my sanity time and again this year and I can't thank you enough for listening to—and responding to—my every thought at all times of the day and night! Thank you to Olivia for just being the best friend anyone could ask for, continually offering such wonderful support and love! Thank you to Matt for always being there for me. And thank you to my awesome friends Oli, Holly, Chloe, India and Imogen for taste-testing so many of these recipes. Although I also have to offer an apology to Oli and Holly for tempting them into eating cake and brownies for breakfast too many times . . .

Thank you to my Deliciously Ella team for keeping me organized and calm. It's been so exciting to watch the company grow and I love being surrounded by such inspiring women every day. It's amazing to work with people who share the same love and passion for healthy living, and your constant energy really keeps me going.

Thank you to Cathryn and Gordy, my incredible agents at WME, for always being so supportive and helpful; there's no way I'd be where I am now without all your wonderful advice. And thanks to Jo, Isabella and Siobhan for all your assistance with absolutely everything.

Thank you to the fantastic team at Hodder who believed in the first book enough to want a second one! With a special thank you to Liz, my brilliant editor, and Eleni, my amazing publicist, for all the enthusiasm you have for Deliciously Ella and for allowing me to share my love of healthy food with the world.

And finally a huge thank you to the amazing team that put this book together—Miranda, Clare, Rosie, Polly, Lucy and Ellie—you are all so incredibly talented and I'm so grateful for all your hard work. You really brought the recipes and the ideas behind Deliciously Ella to life in the most beautiful way.

FOLLOW DELICIOUSLY ELLA

www.deliciouslyella.com

 instagram.com/DeliciouslyElla

 www.facebook.com/Deliciouslyella

 @DeliciouslyElla

 www.youtube.com—search Deliciously Ella

Scribner
An Imprint of Simon & Schuster, Inc.
1230 Avenue of the Americas
New York, NY 10020

For information about special discounts for bulk
purchases, please contact Simon & Schuster
Special Sales at 1-866-506-1949 or
business@simonandschuster.com.

The Simon & Schuster Speakers Bureau can bring
authors to your live event. For more information
or to book an event, contact the Simon & Schuster
Speakers Bureau at 1-866-248-3049 or visit our
website at www.simonspeakers.com.

Manufactured in the United States of America

10 9 8 7 6 5 4 3 2 1

Library of Congress Cataloging-in-Publication
Data is available.

ISBN 978-1-5011-2761-8
ISBN 978-1-5011-2898-1 (ebook)

Design and Art Direction: Miranda Harvey
Photography: Clare Winfield
Editor: Lucy Bannell
Photo Shoot Co-ordinator: Ruth Ferrier
Index: Hilary Bird
Food Stylist: Rosie Reynolds
Assistant Food Stylist: Eleanor Mulligan
Props Stylist: Polly Webb-Wilson
Make-up Artist: Laurey Simmons

With thanks to Anthropologie, Bobbin Bicycles,
Quince (quinceliving.co.uk) and The Glam
Camping Company for generously providing props,
and to Juice Baby for letting us shoot in their store.

Photographs on pages 3, 8, 11, 12, 13, 19, 29, 30,
38, 43, 57, 85, 91, 102, 111, 121, 125, 129, 141, 151,
163, 167, 180, 188, 195, 198, 205, 207, 227, 253
and 256 courtesy of Ella Woodward.

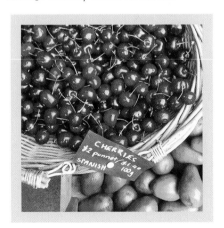